M000206377

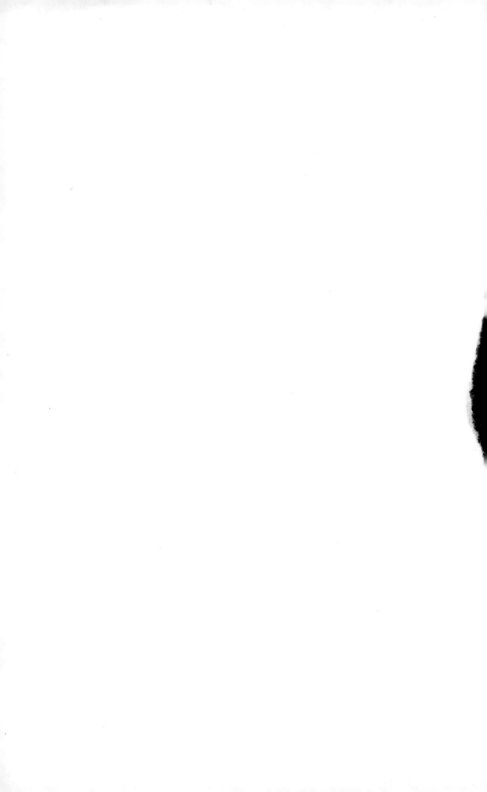

Advance Praise For
Finding a Way

"In *Finding A Way*, Siri doesn't just inspire you to overcome obstacles and live your best life, she teaches you how! She's not just a teacher who knows how to do it, she's a teacher who's actually done it, and that's one in a billion! In *Finding A Way*, Siri gives you the tools to turn the impossible into possible and design the life of your dreams."
— JAMIE KERN LIMA, *New York Times* Bestselling Author of *Believe IT*, and Founder, IT Cosmetics

"In the telling of her heroic journey, Siri Lindley becomes a compass for the reader, a guide on the trail of life, a coach that inspires with clarity and strength for a happier journey."
— MELISSA ETHERIDGE, 2x Grammy Award– and Academy Award–Winning Singer, Songwriter, and Musician

"Want to come home to your truth? Reach for this book. Siri's awe-inspiring journey and loving wisdom will guide your soul to calibrate to your true self."
— LINDA WALLEM, Actress, Writer, Producer, Writer and Producer for *Nurse Jackie*

"Siri is a force of nature; I've never met another person like her. The energy she brings into every single day is unparalleled. But it's her ability to share that energy and use it to lift up those around her that's most admirable. I'm forever grateful for the impact she's had on my life taking me from an average professional triathlete to multiple world champion achieving my every dream along the way."
— MIRINDA CARFRAE, 4x World Champion Triathlete

FINDING A WAY

TAKING THE IMPOSSIBLE AND MAKING IT POSSIBLE

Siri Lindley

Post Hill
PRESS

A POST HILL PRESS BOOK
ISBN: 978-1-63758-792-8
ISBN (eBook): 978-1-63758-793-5

Finding a Way:
Taking the Impossible and Making it Possible
© 2023 by Siri Lindley
All Rights Reserved

Cover design by Conroy Accord
Cover Photo by Erin Cox

Although every effort has been made to ensure that the personal and professional advice present within this book is useful and appropriate, the author and publisher do not assume and hereby disclaim any liability to any person, business, or organization choosing to employ the guidance offered in this book.

This is a work of nonfiction. All people, locations, events, and situation are portrayed to the best of the author's memory.

No part of this book may be reproduced, stored in a retrieval system, or transmitted by any means without the written permission of the author and publisher.

Post Hill Press
New York • Nashville
posthillpress.com

Published in the United States of America
1 2 3 4 5 6 7 8 9 10

"With freedom comes responsibility."
— ELEANOR ROOSEVELT

I have found my way to freedom.
All I want now is to help you find yours.
Through this book I will show you the way.
Each breath I take is a miracle. I feel so
    deeply grateful for this life.
With each breath I strive to love with all my heart, live
    fearlessly, and make a difference in this beautiful world.
This is my gift to you, the reader.

Table of Contents

Foreword by Tony Robbins

There are so many books out there written by individuals who intellectually understand principles. People who can rattle off lists, give lectures, and tell people what to do for a living. If you ever get the chance to meet these folks in person, all too often you may be perplexed to find they're not exactly eating their own cooking, so to speak.

After forty-five years of working with human beings all over the globe, I've trained myself to look for the people who actually live it. The ones that don't just talk a good game but actually walk the walk consistently, earnestly, and authentically in the face of all life has to offer us, even when it's difficult, and even when no one is watching. (Most importantly when it's difficult and especially when no one is watching.)

That's why it delights me to promise you that the book in your hands is a living, breathing testament to the way its author—my dear friend, Siri Lindley—lives her life.

I first met Siri years ago when I called her up on a summer day to interview her as a guest on my podcast. As it turns out, Siri was the first guest interview episode we ever recorded. It came to pass because she and I have a mutual connection; my assistant, Mary, is an old friend of Siri's wife, Rebekah. I remember Mary saying, *"Tony, we'll just record the conversation,*

I know the perfect person, she is a USA Triathlon Hall of Famer, and a former World Champion, etc., etc., BUT, the kicker is, Siri decided she would become the best triathlete even before she knew how to swim! She's a visionary! The best kind of crazy. You'll love her!"

Mary was right. The instant I heard Siri say hello, I fell in love with her love of life.

Siri's exuberance made everyone in the room smile that day. We couldn't help but catch the wave of Siri's joy, grit, honest self-awareness, and relentless optimism. Before we even hung up the phone, I knew our paths were destined to connect, and we have been dear friends ever since.

Make no mistake, though, this is not just another book celebrating athletic triumphs. (She's already written that one.) This is about the human journey and the hero's journey. It's about her determination to focus not on her fear, but rather, on the one thing we all have in common: the gift of this lifetime and what we're going to do with it.

On the phone that day we met, Siri told me that she had been a student of my work for decades. She said she read my old books like *Unlimited Power* and *Awaken the Giant Within*, and she told me how they had impacted her life. The overarching lessons of those books and of the events I host around the world converge on the premise that it's not the conditions of your life, but rather the decisions you make about *what to focus on, what things mean to you, and what you're going to do about them*, that determine your ultimate destiny.

It was clear to me that Siri had absorbed the message and understood the gravitas of those three decisions that we're all making every moment (either consciously or unconsciously). But as I've already said, it's one thing for people to understand something intellectually and quite another rarity to actually DO what they KNOW when the going gets tough.

To understate it, the going got really tough for Siri a few years later. There was another memorable phone call. The one where Siri's wife, Bek, called my wife, Sage, to tell us that Siri had just received a harrowing diagnosis. I'll leave it to Siri to tell you how she found her way—and you can, too—but I will tell you what this woman's journey has meant to me, personally.

The thing about mentorship people don't always talk about is that the river often runs in both directions. I watched—and learned—with great respect and deep honor as Siri decidedly and courageously found her way in the areas that matter most in life—health, family, friends, and fulfillment.

I've had the privilege to learn from many special souls whose mastery of certain areas have provided me with helpful hints about what to anticipate in my own life, people who have navigated the rapids already and are willing to share their hardscrabble map of the territory. I've long suggested that people find those kinds of mentors for themselves, somebody to model, a friend who finds strength in moments of weakness and can offer clear, practical distinctions and proven pathways to power in the face of the inevitable obstacles. Those are the people we all want to listen to. Those are the people who provide a guiding light when we need it most, and that's exactly why Siri's story is so inspiring to me and why it will surely move anyone who goes on this journey with her.

—TONY ROBBINS

PART I
Introduction

You get to go first in deciding what story you want to live.

*I*f the COVID-19 pandemic years have taught us anything, it's not to take anything for granted. Life as we know it can change in a heartbeat—or it can stagnate, leaving us stuck repeating the same unhealthy patterns. I believe I know this better than anyone.

I wanted to be a world champion triathlete—even though I didn't know how to swim. I wanted to love and be loved—even though my hero, my father, shunned me when I told him I was gay. I wanted to rescue horses from slaughter and ban this brutal practice once and for all—even though I only had two years of experience with horses. I wanted to savor every day and enjoy the life I had made with my wife, my career, and my passion for horses and animals—even though in November 2019, I was diagnosed with a rare and usually fatal form of acute myeloid leukemia (AML).

Every time I have been faced with what seemed impossible, I found a way not only to survive the situation but to thrive within it. Today, I am cancer free, a triathlon world champion, happily married, co-founder with my wife of a nonprofit that has rescued 214 horses from slaughter in five years, and one of the most successful coaches and motivational speakers in the world. I overcame the lingering trauma of my childhood and a terrifying bout with crippling obsessive-compulsive disorder (OCD) in my teens and during college, and I have turned it all into a message of hope and love for you.

I am no different than you. You have everything you need inside of you to overcome any challenge and achieve things that seem impossible.

I have suffered deeply for much of my lifetime.

On the outside, my whole life tells a different story: one of overcoming challenges, achieving impossible goals, and being a love and light to all those around me.

This came at a great cost to me internally. I have spent my life wrestling with my fears, keeping my worries to myself, and suffering in silence.

I have been seen as stoic and strong, with superhuman courage and resilience.

My Pandora's box of pain was never revealed to others. I had defined my existence to be one where I must never be a worry. I must never be a problem. I must be the light. I must be the inspiration. I must be the *rock* for everyone around me while also keeping myself standing, holding it together, and finding a way to temper the storm of pain within me. Because of this, I HAD to find a way through my pain, my fear, and my suffering. Because of this desperation, I had no choice but to do everything in my power to find solutions—to find a way.

I am going to share with you the tools and strategies that worked for me through a lot of trial and error and the many times of wanting to give up. By putting them all together in this book, I will help you find a way through your struggles—through them and on to TRIUMPH.

You have everything you need inside of you to do this.

You are the conductor of your own symphony of life.

You get to GO FIRST in deciding what story you want to live in any moment. You get to go first in deciding what is possible for you, what you are capable of, or what any given challenge will mean for you.

It is time to back yourself: stack the proof of all the times you have overcome challenges that seemed insurmountable—all the times you achieved something that seemed impossible.

So often we stack our doubts and fears and that leaves us feeling powerless amid the pain. You don't have to live with this pain and suffering any longer.

Let me teach you how to rewrite the stories in life that you are living. Let me help you re-narrate those stories to bring out your best so you can open the gates to a greener pasture where you can finally put down your armor, open your heart, and receive the gifts of love, joy, and fulfillment that you deserve.

I see you. I feel your pain. I share your fear. I know how to help you through it.

The temporary discomfort you may feel in leaning into this work is way less painful than the long-term suffering you will endure if you continue thinking, believing, and acting in the same ways you have been for so long.

I ask you to trust me and to believe in me. I have weathered all the most harrowing storms. With each storm, however, I was able to come closer to who I am as a human being, what I no longer wanted to experience, and what I know I deserved. First and foremost, this was FREEDOM. Freedom from within.

I will show you how to help yourself: how to free yourself from all that holds you back in your life.

I may be new to this experience of unbridled joy and freedom. I finally felt this freedom, one I have dreamed about for a lifetime, in just the last few years. But, as I trace my steps and unpack the HOW I got here, I feel so compelled—pulled—to share the recipe with you.

You can have the life that you dream of. I don't mean just the successes and accomplishments but finally the fulfillment that you yearn for. The fulfillment and freedom to be: that is the ultimate gift you give yourself.

Finding a Way will guide you through three major principles:

ONE: YOU GET TO CHOOSE WHAT HAPPENS NEXT

I will share stories from my own experiences with cancer, sports, OCD, and coming out to my family as a gay woman to help the reader learn the most important lesson of this book:

> *Whatever you're facing, there is always a way through it, and you have everything you need inside you to find your way.*
>
> *You get to go first in deciding what story you want to live. What meaning do you want to give any challenge? I, Siri, will guide you on how to re-narrate the stories you live to empower and enable you to find a way, not*

*only through the challenges, but TO the life you dream
of living.*

Whether you are facing a decision, a crisis, or a lingering sense of fear and anxiety, I will show you that you can change your own direction, rewrite your story, and define new, more authentic purposes that will help you live the life of your dreams.

What do you want most in your life? What is getting in the way of you having that? Who must you become to live the life you dream of living?

To get to where you want to go, you first need to know who you are. Part 1 guides you through the process of tuning out the outside voices and pressures and focusing instead on discovering your authentic self. What makes you feel alive? What makes you excited to get out of bed in the morning? So often we let ourselves be defined by the expectations of others, but I will show you that we will never find fulfillment if we're trying to live someone else's dreams. Through stories, exercises, and building your own self-awareness, I will help you define your values, listen to your inner voice, and live in alignment with your values, rather than your fear, self-doubt, or anxiety.

TWO: CHANGE YOUR STORY, CHANGE YOUR LIFE

What are the stories that you carry with you? Things from the past often affect how you see yourself in the present, but our stories don't have to be based on the past. Your stories are entirely up to you and how you choose to live in the present. As you make your way through this book, you can take the insights of the Power Line and use them to rewrite your stories, focusing on the things that build you up and carry you toward the future you want for yourself. We'll explore how you can use your strengths, your values, and all that time you've already used to overcome a lifetime of negative messaging. I will show you how to "stack your proof," preparing for the days when you have setbacks or doubts and moving forward seems impossible.

THREE: FINDING A WAY WITH THE POWER LINE

As I traced back the steps in my life that have led me to find a way through every challenge, I discovered the key elements that I embodied to succeed. You have all of these within you already. It's a matter of deciding to lead with these things to show up prepared for the road ahead.

Choosing to be INTENTIONAL with these things is what will get you from being someone who has, for example, courage, to being courageous.

You will learn how to dig deep to bring out these practices in your life and condition them so they become your strongest attributes. It will enable you to find a way through any challenge and achieve things that may, at some point, seem impossible.

Each chapter will explore one of these key attributes that you need to live the life that reflects your values and your dreams.

- The power of Going First
- The power Identity and Authenticity
- The power of Courage

- The power of Gratitude
- The power of Intention
- The power of Presence
- The power of Purpose
- The power of Forgiveness
- The power of the Unexpected Teacher
- The power of Decisions
- The power of Resilience
- The power of Health
- The power of Faith
- The power of Love

Ultimately, the message of this book comes back to love, and in particular, the importance of loving yourself, trusting yourself, and backing yourself. You must give yourself permission to live the best life possible.

Every breath in life is a miracle.

One of the most profound gifts I received through my fight with leukemia was a commitment to myself that I would live every moment ON PURPOSE, celebrating all the gifts of who I am in every moment. I loved myself, believed in myself, and was present in as many moments as possible.

As I lay in my hospital bed faced with the possibility of death, I began thinking about whether I would feel as though I lived life to the fullest. I realized three questions that will matter most to me at the end of my days:

1. Did I live fully and fearlessly?
2. Did I love with all my heart? Others and me?
3. Did I make a difference? In other words, did I matter?

I feel so deeply blessed to have the opportunity to ensure that I answer those questions in the affirmative. It is my responsibility to do this FOR ME.

Life is short. We don't know how long we have on this planet. What will matter most to you?

Are you living life to reflect that?

I will help you do just that.

I believe in you. I want you to live the life you dream of— to free yourself from the shackles that have held you back from the joy and love you deserve. We are in this together.

By the end of this book, you will know how to rewrite the stories from your past that have been holding you back. It will light the path for you to truly live life on purpose and experience all that you want in life.

You will have the tools to overcome your anxiety and see fear as your friend.

You will find your way home to YOU. Your authentic self. With that, you will find your FREEDOM!

TOOLS AND RESOURCES:

This is not just a book of motivational stories and ideas. I take the insights and lessons of *Finding a Way* and turn them into practical, applicable exercises to help you use them in your life. These will include questions to consider on their own, conversations to conduct with others, and practical actions to take in support of your changes. I am with you every step of the way, and together we will celebrate at the end.

Chapter 1

I CHOSE TO LIVE

I thought I was going to the hospital for a hip replacement. After thirty years of pushing my body as an athlete, including eight years where I trained way beyond my capabilities to be the best triathlete in the world, my body needed replacement parts.

Choosing triathlon was my way of minimizing the emotional pain I was fraught with. Because I pushed so hard in training and was able to withstand so much pain, it distracted me from my emotions. This eased my suffering.

Thus, I had trained like a maniac for eight years, beyond what my body was capable of. By training hard, my pain became external, easier to handle than the internal storm of anxiety, fear, loss, and abandonment.

A few hours after my pre-op appointment, a nurse told me we needed to postpone the surgery because there was something weird in my bloodwork. They referred me to specialists at the University of Colorado Anschutz Medical Campus outside of Denver, who brought me in for a full day of testing, including a painful bone marrow biopsy and a spinal tap.

Two days before Thanksgiving, my doctor called with the test results. I put him on speakerphone so that Bek, my wife, could hear his report with me.

While Bek was standing with me at our kitchen counter, my doctor delivered the horrifying diagnosis. "Siri, you have acute myeloid leukemia with a genetic mutation that is going to make this very complicated to treat."

My wife started wailing. Tears poured down her face. My doctor's voice shook. I remember objectively taking in everything going on around me. The resounding message I was hearing was "this is the end."

I felt a wave of devastation coursing through every part of my body: a terror.

Shock. Sadness. I have never been so afraid in my entire life.

My doctor's words cut me like a knife. My greatest fear was now my reality. The sense of terror, loss of my life: finally, what I had worked for a lifetime to create was now seemingly being taken away from me. Finally, I had love. Finally, I had a purpose and a mission outside of just freeing myself from my internal pain. I had a career I loved, and I felt safe in my own skin. It was a lifelong dream of mine. But now, I was not safe in this body. Now, this disease was threatening to take it all away. The depth of that pain is indescribable. The fear I felt, paralyzing.

Shaking myself out from being frozen in fear, I made the most powerful decision of my entire life.

THIS IS NOT MY TIME TO GO. I am going to survive, and I am going to THRIVE.

I am NOT a statistic. I am SIRI LINDLEY, and I chose to live on that day.

Coming to terms with the diagnosis was not easy, but I knew that to survive I had to change the way I looked at it. I had to remember who I was, what I had achieved, and what I was capable of.

I had to GO FIRST in deciding what story I was going to live. This could NOT be the end. This had to be the beginning. It was a challenge that would help me become who I needed to be to truly live this life at the level I was destined to.

This AML did not come to destroy me. It came to free me.

There's a saying I've thought about a lot since that day: "Everything you are going through now is preparing you for what you asked for." Those words rang true to me as soon as I heard them, but also left me wondering: had I asked for cancer to come into my life?

In my twenties, I found triathlon. I was desperate to find appreciation and love for myself after realizing I was gay and losing my father because of it. I had to take on something that seemed impossible. I had to take on something that would allow me to channel my devastation over losing my father's love and my anxiety and fear of what life would now become.

This was the vehicle through which I would find myself and hopefully find a way to love and respect myself regardless of my sexual orientation.

This was my escape vehicle. This was my RIDE OR DIE.

I fell in love with the sport of triathlon, watching a friend compete in one. I didn't know how to swim, and I was already twenty-three years old, but in watching the myriad of people taking on the challenge, I just knew I had to do one.

In my first race, I came in dead last. I embarrassed myself by getting in a lane way too fast for me, getting in everyone else's way, and running with my bike helmet on.

Regardless, I had never felt so alive in my entire life.

I decided on the eve of that first race that I was going to be the best in the world in the sport one day.

Crazy. Yes, I know. But I had a deep emotional reason WHY I had to do this for myself: I had to find an appreciation for myself, respect for myself, and love for myself.

This was my journey, and I would do everything I could to make myself proud.

I was doing something for myself. It was something I needed to break free from the prison I held myself in.

I immersed myself in the sport. It determined where I lived and how I spent my time, twenty-four hours a day and seven days a week. I lived, ate, slept, and breathed triathlon.

In taking on this impossible dream, I realized two things had to happen.

With any great goal, I encourage you to ask yourself these two questions:

What do I need to let go of to achieve this goal? And who do I need to become?

I needed to let go of trying to be everything I thought I needed to be for everyone around me. I needed to be fearlessly, authentically me. This is how I could truly tap into everything I had inside of me that could help me make this happen.

I needed to become someone willing to fail. I needed to understand that it is through our failures, through our disappointments, that we learn and grow the most. This is HOW we make progress—the progress necessary to ultimately achieve the goal we set for ourselves.

If you are not willing to fail, you are not willing to succeed.

So, I changed the meaning of both success and failure.

Success was progress, being better than I was the day before, whether that be physically, mentally, or emotionally. BETTER was success.

Success was being the best me that I could be every single day.

Failure was LEARNING. It was a necessary part of becoming who I needed to become to achieve my impossible dream.

Every day, I was either winning or I was learning. This served me well.

The Olympic trials were the be-all, end-all for me. It was everything I had set my heart upon for six years. But I choked on the big day after sacrificing EVERYTHING I knew for this one goal. I choked and then swiftly lost total control over my emotions and my focus. I quit, and I pulled out of the race. I felt like a complete failure by proving my biggest fear that I would never be enough.

I wanted to climb into a hole and never come out. Shame buried me, not offering a crack of light to see any hope for my future.

When in deep depression, it is so hard to see any way out. Sometimes it takes someone else coming and shaking you hard to wake you up to the truth. They get you to stop obsessing over your own pain and focus on something outside of yourself.

That person for me was Loretta Harrop, who would ultimately become my most profound competitor and best friend.

In a world where I felt so invisible, she saw me, she felt my pain, and she put out her hand to help me out of the hole I was in. She offered me to join her training squad, coached by Brett Sutton.

Brett Sutton was the best coach in the world. He coached world champions and Olympic medalists, and I wanted him to coach me.

When I finally got in front of him, he looked at me and said, "I remember you. I was walking home from a race. All my athletes had already finished. But you were still running. You were in something like twenty-ninth place, and you were *absolutely killing yourself* to get to twenty-eighth." He nodded. "I like that. It's hunger." And amazingly, he agreed to coach me.

I moved to Switzerland to be in his training camp, and it took me about five minutes to realize I was absolutely the *worst* athlete there. I was the slowest at everything. But Brett didn't give me a break. He demanded that I dive right into his brutal training schedule of six to eight hours every day, right alongside the women and men who were already world champions. It felt almost inhumane, and I called my mom almost every night in tears.

After eight days of that, I couldn't move my arms or my legs. I hobbled over to Brett and confessed, "I don't think I can do what you're asking me to do today. I can't move." I waved my arms weakly to show him how much pain I felt.

But Brett didn't look at my arms. He barely looked at me at all as he shrugged. "Find a way," he said.

Find a way.

All I could do was the best that I could with what I had and try to find a way.

It was brilliant because every single day he was giving me something that seemed IMPOSSIBLE. But I just did the best that I could and proved to myself that what seems impossible is possible.

How can you ever know what you are truly capable of if you don't try something that you don't think you can do, every single day? You must get out of your comfort zone—live there even.

Live there I did.

The depth of suffering we went to each day in training was magnified by my loud and obnoxious voice of anxiety that seemed to make every effort even harder due to my fear of failure and not being enough.

Thus, the emotional toll was almost harder to bear than the physical. The more tired I got, the harder it was to handle my fear and anxiety. But I had no choice. I had to find a way.

I stayed in Brett's agonizing, punishing training program for two solid years, and in that time, I won thirteen Triathlon World Cup races, two World Championships, (Triathlon World Championships 2001 and Aquathon World Championship 2001) two world titles, and retired as the number one ranking triathlete in the world.

The most profound reward: finding love and appreciation for myself. Finally. This is what mattered most.

I had proved to myself that I could count on myself. I could believe in myself. I could love myself.

The other profound gift was a shift in my identity. I had formed a new identity, one that served me beautifully in everything that came my way in the future. I WILL ALWAYS FIND A WAY.

Through any pain, through any challenge, through any struggle, I knew I could survive. I knew I had everything I needed inside of me to overcome.

The inner strength this takes is beyond comprehension. It always felt like such a push—SUCH HARD WORK. My dream was to, one day, achieve with more flow, not force.

In dedicating myself to figuring out how to do this, I had to try on different mindsets. I had to master the skill of reframing to empower myself in any situation. I had to condition new patterns of thought, focus, and meaning.

I had to learn how to recognize the stories that held me back in life: the stories that caused me pain, suffering, and fear.

All that I learned led me to TRIUMPH over acute myeloid leukemia. It was a miracle. I AM A MIRACLE.

All the tools I used to get me through the darkest times in my life, I am now going to give to you.

All I want to do now is help free you from the force, the pain, and the suffering. I want to help you find a better way.

It's a way that takes care of you, supports you, and allows you to truly live life at the highest levels.

Why should you trust me? My lifetime has been the playing field on which I have created my strategy for FINDING A WAY. In peeling back the layers of my life, I have been able to recognize the formula that led me to my freedom and my success.

In college, I almost took my own life due to my debilitating OCD. It was my way of managing the overwhelming anxiety and fear I felt. No one spoke of fear or anxiety, nor about behaviors like flicking lights on and off for thirty minutes until you got a horrible thought out of your mind. No one EVER discussed these things, so I thought I was the ONLY person in the world who felt them. So alone, I couldn't handle it anymore. Thank God, this is when Tony Robbins's teachings came into my life. He woke me to the TRUTH that the only person that could save me was me.

Was I worth saving? Was I willing to participate in my own rescue? I had no choice. This led me to choose psychology as a major because I was desperate to figure out why I suffered as I did and wanted to try to find a solution.

My father, my hero, cut me out of his life when he found out I was gay. This broke me into a million pieces. The person I loved the most was telling me I was worthless—not just worthless but an embarrassment to him. Where did that leave me? ALONE. ABANDONED. WORTHLESS. DESPERATE to somehow find worthiness from within.

IT WAS ALL UP TO ME.

I was FORCED to learn all the tools and strategies I will share with you in this book. It was that or die.

I am thankful now that I had to go through all that pain because it made me who I am today. It gave me PURPOSE!

I want to free you from the pain that I know all too well. I want to help you find a way out of the storm that never seems to subside.

WHY ME?

In the years since I retired from triathlon competitions, my goals and my purpose had changed. As a coach, an animal advocate, a speaker, and a wife, what I asked for now was to touch as many lives as possible in beautiful and powerful ways. I was living the life of my dreams, and I wanted everyone else to have that, too, so all I asked was to share my experiences so that others could find the same beautiful and powerful magic inside themselves.

I'd been through plenty of things that seemed to connect with people. I'd decided to become a world champion triathlete—and I did it. Before that, in college, I'd decided to overcome my crippling OCD—and I did it. I'd decided to forgive and rebuild a relationship with my father after he shunned me for years—and I did it. More recently, Bek and I decided to launch a local rescue and national advocacy program for horses bound for slaughter—and we did it.

Thinking about all of that always brought tears to my eyes, but as I settled into a deep gratitude for this life I was living, I also found myself thinking about how there was still so much more that I wanted to learn about myself and about life. I was being invited to speak on these big stages, next to these people I'd admired all my life, and sometimes I wondered: did I deserve to be there? After all, lots of people had incredible success stories. Why did mine matter?

And then I received a devastating, possibly fatal cancer diagnosis that brought me to my knees. I had to give it an empowering meaning. I had to believe that it happened for a greater purpose.

A focus on "why me?" would not equip me with the mind-set and energy necessary to beat this. I needed to tell a different story and give it a different meaning. What if this was another time where "what I am going through now is preparing me for what I asked for"?

What did I ask for? Well, I had been feeling this deep and powerful pull to want to touch lives and make a beautiful difference in this world. Maybe who I would become through this challenge would be the person that could do that on a larger scale. I would learn things about myself, about finding a way through great challenges that could help others do the same.

So, in the days and weeks after my diagnosis, I chose to see this leukemia as the thing that would prepare me for what I asked for.

I chose to look at the cancer that had invaded my life and see it as a gift.

I had to. This was the only meaning that would strengthen me, not destroy me.

During the years when I was in my prime fitness and training for triathlons, some of the hardest times, mentally, would come when I'd get a running injury that would keep me off my feet and away from my training regimen. Here I was, gearing up for these big events, and I was literally hobbled. There was nothing I could do but stay off my feet and wait to heal.

At first, those times seemed like the end of the world, but Brett never let me wallow. I couldn't run, he'd tell me, but I could still swim and bike. In fact, I could swim and bike *more* and *longer* because I couldn't run. And since the swim was always my absolute weakness, and my biking still definitely needed help, putting in that extra time in those areas brought me closer to what I asked for. I wanted to be the best in the world in triathlon, and I succeeded.

There was a gift in my struggle.

Wait. This is important. Please read that again.

There is a gift in every struggle.

Cancer was the gift that would give me a deeper understanding of myself. It showed me what I truly wanted in life, what mattered most, and what was necessary to live the life I dreamed of. I then could share all these discoveries with others to help them navigate their own lives.

I just had to find a way through it.

I didn't let myself wallow in my diagnosis or focus on the worst-case outcome. Instead, supported by my "A-Team" of Bek and my mom, I dove right in because I understood that surviving and thriving wasn't going to just happen to me. It was something I needed to *make* happen.

That's important enough to repeat, too.

If you want something to happen, don't wait for it. Make it happen.

Almost on the same day that Bek and I first heard the phrase "acute myeloid leukemia," we learned that my hospital, UCHealth Anschutz, was starting a new clinical trial for a new type of targeted treatment for cancer like mine. Just a few days later, I signed up to be the seventh person *ever* to receive the treatment. There was more bloodwork, more painful bone marrow biopsies, and a two-week stay in the hospital while I took a regimen of antiviral medication.

By January, the drugs had pushed my leukemia into a short-term remission, and the doctor who would handle my bone marrow transplant, Dr. Jonathan Gutman, called and told me I needed to come to the hospital right away for the next phase of treatment. "We are going to have to drop the biggest bomb on you that your body can handle, right before it kills you," he said. To give the new bone marrow cells the best chance to save my life, he had to basically destroy my immune system so that my body wouldn't reject the transplant.

"It's going to be rough," he told me in his dry, understated way.

But this was what was needed for me to live, so I went back to UCHealth in February for a week of intensive chemotherapy and radiation and remained there through March to receive a bone marrow transplant, which included cells donated by my sister. The procedure was paired up with donated umbilical cord stem cells that could grow new cells quickly while decreasing my body's chances of cell rejection or infection.

Dr. Gutman was right about bringing me right to the edge. In those weeks, I was sick in a way I'd never been before, and it was THE hardest time—physically, emotionally, and mentally—of my entire life.

I had to constantly discipline my focus in every single moment to keep myself from falling apart and giving up.

I don't know what I would have done without my mom, who gave up everything in her life for more than a month to sleep on the couch in my hospital room, and yet she remained constantly cheerful. This all happened just as the COVID-19 pandemic was spreading across the country, and so I was separated from Bek, who had to quarantine after an event out of state, and from my beloved animals. I fell into a deep depression and hit a very dark time inside myself. The pain was more than I'd ever felt. I could feel the cancer testing me at the core of my identity, robbing me of my strength and bringing up fears that shook me to the bone.

I would catch myself in those rock-bottom moments where I was obsessing over my sickness, pain, sadness, and fear. I would say, "Siri, focusing on how bad you feel and how sick you are is NOT going to help you heal. It's only going to make you feel worse. So, I would change the channel. To GRATITUDE."

I had gratitude for the incredible doctors and nurses working tirelessly to save my life; gratitude for my incredible mom who never left my side; gratitude for Bek, the love of my life, for bringing me strength, love, and inspiration; and gratitude for my sister and the umbilical cord that were giving me life!

GRATITUDE WAS THE BRIDGE FROM DESPAIR TO HOPE.

Gratitude gave me energy. Gratitude gave me hope. Gratitude was the answer and always is.

In times of great despair, you must refrain from stacking your doubts and fears. Instead, stack your proof!

I had a poster on my hospital wall of me winning the World Triathlon Championships—my impossible dream coming true. That was my proof. It was proof of WHO I AM and proof that what seems impossible is possible.

YOU have proof also: proof of the times you overcame a challenge that seemed insurmountable, proof of the times you achieved something you didn't think you could.

In times of deep despair, stack your proof NOT your doubts.

In April, I was finally discharged and allowed to go home to my wife and my animals, and they surrounded me with love and healing. I rejoiced in every small moment—walking outside with my mom, riding my horse Savannah, holding my wife's hand. I was struck hard with digestion issues that were my body's reaction to the new immune system that had taken over.

I would sometimes get so very sick, vomiting over thirty times in one day.

It was my worst nightmare. Throughout my life, my biggest phobia was vomiting. Now, I was faced with it nearly every day.

I was on like seventy-five different tablets a day, and my body was responding as if it were under threat. I kept telling myself, "This is saving me. This is giving me life."

I would pray before taking every tablet: "Thank you. Thank you for bringing me back to life." Again, it was a way to reframe the medication not as poison but as something that was saving my life.

My wife had to clean out my PICC (peripherally inserted central catheter) line every day. This was a full-on medical procedure, but she learned how to do it and never complained.

Bek would have to cover my lines with saran wrap before every shower as I couldn't get it wet. She never complained. She was my superhero.

I started worrying about her falling out of love with me. There I was, asking her to do these very difficult things. I was throwing up countless times a day and weak. I was bald, sick, and unable to do all the things I used to do around the house, with the horses, and in my life.

I would look at myself in the mirror, skinny and weak, and be consumed with the thought that Bek would leave me because I was no longer the person she fell in love with. Despite seeing those tears in her eyes, despite her daily encouragement and assurances, my heart still believed she loved me only because of what I could achieve. I thought she was attracted to my physical strength and all the energy that I poured into her and into others. I thought she loved my accomplishments. Now I couldn't perform the most basic tasks for myself, and I needed to be taken care of in ways that were often embarrassing. If I didn't look strong or fit, if I didn't have the energy to do all the things we loved doing together, if I couldn't achieve anything or impress her, why would she stay?

Bek stayed, of course, because she loved me—ME, not what I looked like or the things I did. Bek loves my heart, my soul, and my spirit, just as I love hers. She saw, even on my weakest days, that I was still me. I wouldn't have seen that without cancer.

I, for fifty years of my life, had been believing my worthiness and lovability lay in my accomplishments, what I could do for others, my energy, and my passion.

The most powerful discovery through this was that my worthiness has nothing to do with those things. That was just a story I have told myself for a lifetime. I was worthy because of how deeply I loved, how much I cared, and who I was on the inside.

This was so liberating.

In May 2020, I had another bone marrow biopsy, and it showed I was cancer free.

What a miracle, an absolute miracle. I felt so deeply grateful, so deeply blessed. So relieved.

There are so many struggles in the world, and in life, right now that can seem like they're impossible to get through. At one point or another, most of us face big, hard questions. Maybe that's what brought you to this book. You're feeling stuck in some part of your life, and the breakthroughs just aren't coming.

Every day, I talk to people like you, who are asking the big questions.

I have a dream that seems impossible. How can I make it happen?

I am faced with a giant obstacle on my path. How can I overcome it?

I live with anger and resentment caused by someone who hurt me deeply. How can I overcome this?

I feel like I've been treading water and going nowhere. How can I live a more fulfilling life?

It's been a hard year. How can I find joy again?

How can I find purpose in my life?

How come I can never seem to get out of my own way?

Those are tough situations, but what I've come to understand is that there's something tougher than all those things, and that something is you.

Whatever you're facing, there is always a way.

And you have everything inside you to find and follow it.

I used to wake up in the morning and think, "I hope it's going to be a good day." Before a race, I would send a prayer out to the universe, "I hope I get to have a good race." It sounded nice, but the reality was that I was passing my power off to something else, not understanding that what happened wasn't up to some outside force beyond my control. It was up to *me*, and only me, to have a good day, or a good race.

It was up to me to treat cancer not as a death sentence but as a gift, and to use the circumstance to move toward the things I wanted to experience in the world.

What is it that you want to experience? What do you want to move toward? What do you want to move past?

Whatever it is, you can do it.

You are so much more powerful than you could ever imagine. Cancer showed me that we have everything we need inside us, all the time. Sometimes it's hard to believe that because it's scary to think about what we're capable of. Sometimes it seems like a lot of responsibility. But I'm living proof that the impossible is really possible—not just in sports, but in life.

Yes, seeking your way every day will be hard sometimes. You'll face challenges. Things will get uncertain. You're going to be afraid, but that doesn't have to stop you. Because all those things that you're dreaming of right now are possible. The solutions to the problems that keep you awake at night are in your hands. It's up to you. You can find a way—your own way—through whatever it is. You can change your direction, rewrite your story, refocus your attention, and live the life of your dreams.

In the pages that follow we will journey together to overcome the things that hold you back, whether it's fear, perfectionism, anxiety, self-doubt, or simply lack of clarity. We'll chart a path—a Power Line—to the life you are longing to live. Because I'm a coach, and I love making training programs, you'll find exercises at the end of most chapters to help you take an idea and put it into practice. Saddle up; it's going to be a lot. This book contains everything I know at this point in my life, and it's something I hope you come back to time after time. Living fully, deeply, and authentically isn't something you will learn overnight. But with each chapter, I'm going to give you a new insight into how you can live the life you want. Each page will get you one step closer.

You get to choose what happens next—how you will read this book, and how you will approach your life.

Not me. Not your parents. Not your spouse or your boss or that person on Facebook who looks like they have the life you want.

Only you.

You get to choose whether to tap into your personal power and give yourself permission to trust yourself. You get to choose how you respond and how you react to everything that happens. You get to choose whether the thing that's in front of you will bring you to your knees or whether you will rise above it.

You can find peace. You can find fulfillment. You can turn your struggle into a gift.

I believe that in the deepest part of my heart. I believe that everything I've been through, from the challenges of my childhood to the long hours I spent in that hospital bed, showed me how to live fully. They taught me how to find joy. And now I want to give that knowledge away, to you. I can't just hold it inside of myself. That's not why it happened. I want you to feel the way I do. I want you to live the life of your dreams. I want to help you let go of the self-doubt, fear, and anxiety that's paralyzing you, and I want to show you how to open yourself to something entirely new.

That may seem scary. You may not think you're capable of doing this.

I know that you are.

You can find a way through what you're facing, too. You can take what seems impossible and make it possible.

When you understand who you are, unburden yourself from the expectations and responsibilities that others have placed on you, and focus on where you're going instead of where you've been, you can create a new story for yourself. When you stop comparing yourself to others, you can be the best you that you can be.

It's not an easy process. There's work to be done. Just as you can be the champion of your own life and create a masterpiece out of anything, you can also be your own worst enemy and orchestrate a tragedy. But as we start this journey together, here's what I want you to know most of all: it's up to you.

What's holding you back? Only yourself.

Let's unravel those ties together. Let's craft new stories, new habits, and new perspectives that will allow you to make what seems impossible right now into something possible.

Remember:

- "Everything you are going through now is preparing you for what you asked for."

- In times of deep despair stack your proof NOT your doubts.

- Gratitude is the bridge from despair to hope.

- You are so much more powerful than you could ever imagine.

- To find out what you are capable of, you must do what you don't think you can.

- There is a gift in every struggle.

ASSIGNMENT: PERSONAL VALUES

Here we will identify your personal values: what is most important to you in your life. Our values influence what we do, how we think, and how we feel about the world around us. When we do or see things that go against our values, we feel bad. We are sad, angry, or disappointed.

When we live in alignment with our values, we feel great—we're authentic, fulfilled, and happy!

Knowing your values gives you a moral compass. Your top values reveal what drives and inspires you. Your values show you what you want in life and will show you what you should move toward and what you should move away from.

Once you know your top values, you can make more informed decisions in life. You will better be able to choose jobs, activities, and friends that support and enhance your values—and avoid those that contradict them.

Values often change over time, so I encourage you to do this exercise annually.

For example, if you're training for a triathlon or trying to get pregnant, "health" is most likely your top value.

But if you're going back to school, or taking on a new position, then growth and learning might be one of your top values! Because our values can change over time, we can find ourselves outgrowing a certain job or position or the friends we used to hang out with.

Put the time and effort into this exercise, and you will see just how valuable this information will be for you in living a life that truly fulfills you.

Write a list of about twenty to thirty things that matter most to you!

Just brainstorm and get it all out on paper.

Don't judge your choices, just come from your heart.

- Think about times you have been happy, alive, and content. This usually signifies your values being met.
- Think about times when you were unhappy, angry, disappointed, or unfulfilled. This usually signifies unmet values.

Next Step: Review and Condense

Look at your long list of values. Let's put similar items in groups and then pick out the one that pulls at you the most. For example:

HEALTH/fitness, strength, endurance

INTEGRITY/trust, honesty, truth.

Choose ten top values.

My Top 10 Values

1.

2.

3.

4.

5.

6.

7.

8.

9.

10.

Now, let's prioritize your top ten.

Be patient and set aside some time to do this. This is the most important part.

Knowing your true top ten values in order will give you a much clearer perspective on why your life is the way it is. What is missing? What needs to change? What is working?

Use this system to prioritize your top values:

1. At first sight, prioritize your values. Number them one to ten.
2. Now, take the first value (1) on your list below and compare it to the second item (2). Do this by answering this question below:

"If I had to choose between having (1) and NOT (2),

OR having (2) and NOT (1) for the rest of my life—which would it be?"

Think carefully! **Use your heart to choose mindfully.**

1. If (1) wins, compare (1) to the next item (3) on your list. Use the same question: "Would I rather have (1) and NOT (3), or (3) and NOT (1) for the rest of my life?"
2. Keep working your way down the list until an item beats (1).
3. If you get to the bottom of your list and nothing beats (1), then (1) is your top value. Write (1) in the number one spot in your prioritized values list and start the process again with (2).
4. However, if an item, say (4), beats (1), simply continue the question process down the list using the new "most important'" value of (4). Continue from (5)—if (1) beat all the items above, then (4) will too!
5. If you get to the bottom of the list and nothing beats (4), then (4) is your top value: Write (4) in the number one spot in your Top Values List.
6. Then return to (1) and repeat the process down the list (from (5) forward) to see if anything else beats (1).
7. If (1) now beats all your other values, it is your second-most important value. Place it in the number two spot.

8. Repeat this process until you have a prioritized order for your values.

My Initial Top 10 Values

1.

2.

3.

4.

5.

6.

7.

8.

9

10.

My Final Prioritized Top 10 Values

1.

2.

3.

4.

5.

6.

7.

8.

9.

10.

Now that you have your top ten life values, here are some questions that will guide you to use this golden information to change your life for the better.

1. What did you learn about yourself during this values exercise?
2. Were there any big surprises?
3. What could you do differently to align yourself more powerfully with your top values?
4. What could you do more of?
5. What could you stop doing?
6. What could you do less of?
7. What could you start doing?
8. What must you continue doing?
9. What is something you can do every single day to live in alignment with your top values?
10. What MUST you have in your life to be happy and fulfilled?

11. What must you avoid to be happy and fulfilled?
12. What do you want most in your life?
13. How important will it be for you to live in alignment with your top values to achieve that?
14. What have the consequences been of NOT living in alignment with the values that matter most to you?
15. What will the consequences be in the future if you continue not living in alignment?
16. If you live in alignment with your top values, what will life look like in the next five years?

PART 2
The Power Line

To deliver this book to you, I needed to go back in time and figure out what my recipe for success was— my recipe for overcoming challenges, for achieving the impossible.

What is the area of your life that you are happy with? That you feel is going well?

That you feel you have found success?

What in your life is good right now? What makes it good? Why are you happy with it?

What made it work?

How have you made it successful? What is/was your strategy for success?

What had to happen to achieve success in this area of your life?

What ingredients were required in creating this success?

I am going to share what I believe are the key ingredients to finding a way through any challenge and achieving any great goal you set your mind to. They are what I call THE POWER LINE.

Chapter 2

THE POWER OF GOING FIRST

The first, most important tool I want to share with you is how to GO FIRST in deciding what is possible for you. Go FIRST in deciding what you are capable of. Go FIRST in deciding what any given challenge will mean to you.

YOU are the conductor of your own life's symphony.

If you don't like the music you are creating, you are the ONLY one who has the power to change it.

You get to go first in deciding what to focus on in life.

Are you focusing on what is missing? Or on what you have?

Are you focusing on what is wrong? Or what is right?

Are you focusing on the problems? Or all possible solutions?

Are you focusing on everything you fear? Or don't want to have happen?

Or are you focusing on what you love and want to create in your life?

Are you focusing on what you have no control over—other people, what they do, how they respond, and how they react?

Or are you focusing on what you have ALL the control over—your own experience of life in every single moment, how you respond, how you react, and the meaning you give everything that happens?

What we decide to focus on and the meaning we give things that happen will determine how deeply we will suffer in life or how free we can become—free to find joy, inner peace, and independence in our internal worlds.

As my greatest mentor, Tony Robbins, said, "Where focus goes, energy flows."

What you focus on grows. Focus on all the bad, you will attract worse.

Focus on all the good, you will attract better.

It's simple but so very powerful.

In college, I was desperate to escape the volatile battlefield of my own mind. I was stuck in a thought cycle that locked me away in an internal prison. I was trying to be everything I thought I needed to be for everyone else around me.

All I knew was that if I achieved, if I was never a worry, if I was everything that I knew would make my family happy, then the chances of my losing them became less and less.

The problem was that I was losing myself. Entirely.

I had no idea who I was.

Once I realized that my life was UP TO ME, I went first in deciding that I would no longer live this story that was making my life feel like a fight for survival in every moment.

Consciously, I gave myself permission to accept the truth that life was up to me.

If I wanted to get out of this self-made prison, I had to shift my thinking.

I used the same discipline that I used every day to get to class, study hard, practice hard, and take care of my body to thrive as a three-sport varsity athlete and successful student.

I needed to channel that same discipline into my focus.

I had to develop an awareness for recognizing when I was focusing on something that was causing me pain or suffering and immediately CHANGE THE CHANNEL.

I had to discipline myself to focus on what I had: my health, a great education, athleticism, and a family that loved me.

I had to focus on what I loved and wanted to create: happiness, internal peace, and becoming the best athlete I could be. I wanted to learn as much as I could to better understand myself and find love and acceptance.

I constantly reminded myself that LIFE WAS UP TO ME.

This freed me from the chains of my OCD and led me to a deep desire to want to find out who I was.

What did I want in life?

What inspired me?

What mattered to me?

I needed to explore my own beliefs. Were they serving me? Or were they holding me back from everything I wanted in life?

Further, are your beliefs your own? Or did you adopt the beliefs of your parents or teachers growing up?

Remember:

- Life is up to you.

- What we decide to focus on and the meaning we give things that happen will determine how deeply we will suffer in life or how free we can become.

ASSIGNMENT: PATTERNS OF THOUGHT AND BELIEFS

Let's take a moment to explore your patterns of focus and beliefs.

Often, we don't know why we are suffering or why we can't seem to get out of our own way.

Building awareness about your internal patterns will help shed some light on those things that must change to move forward.

Think about how much time you spend thinking about the following.

Pay attention to your answers and ask yourself, "Is this helping me live the life I want to live? Or is it holding me back or causing me pain?"

Focus Patterns

Negative

What is missing?

What is wrong?

What are my problems?

What do I have no control over?

What do I fear?

What about the past and any pain I endured?

What do I worry about for the future?

How far I must go?

Positive

What do I have?

What is right?

What are possible solutions?

What do I love?

What do I want to create?

What do I have control over?

How am I in the present moment?

How far have I come?

How do you see these patterns affecting your experience of life?

What is your prevailing state of being?

Is it frazzled, anxious, depressed, or overwhelmed? Or are you happy, calm, and poised?

What do you notice about your focus and how it affects your experience of life?

Goal for this week and beyond:

In any moment where you catch yourself focusing on what is missing, what is wrong, or what you have no control over—STOP and pause.

Ask yourself, "What can I be grateful for in this moment? What can I appreciate in this moment?"

This will be the stimulus for you to change the channel and redirect your focus to what is right, what you have, what you can control, and the present moment where you can make better choices, better decisions, protect yourself from pain, and open yourself up to joy.

Chapter 3

THE POWER OF STORY

CHANGE YOUR STORY TO CHANGE YOUR LIFE

You get to GO FIRST in deciding what story in life you want to live.

With each of the greatest challenges in life, I had to go first in deciding what that challenge would mean to me. What story in life did I want to live?

For example, let's go back to my college days. Here I was debilitated emotionally by my OCD. I was terrified in my own skin, exhausted from trying to hide it all, and feeling so desperately alone. What turned me around ultimately was my decision that I DID NOT want to live this story—this tragedy. I refused to let this be my present and my future.

I had to decide to write a new story. It would be one that reflected what I wanted most in life: inner peace. I wanted to know myself. I wanted to feel safe in my own skin. I wanted to love myself and enjoy life—not live in fear and suffering.

The story I was living was "I am crazy." I do these things that I am so ashamed of. No one knows the real me. I don't know if I have what it takes to live another day.

This story had to change if I were to one day find that inner peace, love for myself, and love for life.

My new story became "I am the only person that has the power to change my experience of life. I choose to live a story of triumph and self-discovery. I choose to live a story where I am the hero and the victor, not the victim."

So, what had to happen for me to believe that I could be THAT person?

I needed to condition this new story by creating a role model in this "future me."

What would THAT person do in this moment?

Would she focus on everything that was wrong with her and that was missing? Would she focus on how far she had to go to get that peace she so desperately yearned for?

NO!!

The "future me" would focus on everything that was right, everything she had, and how far she had come in the process of freeing herself from her own pain.

What would that "future me" do?

Would she continue to do the things she was doing? NO!

The "future me" would learn more about what I was experiencing.

She would commit to disciplining her focus to empower herself, not weaken herself.

The "future me" would set out on a mission to discover who she really is, what she wants, the things she loves, and set goals to move closer to what she wants her life to be.

Looking back, I have been able to see what my process was. I wanted to figure this out so that I can share it with you and so that you can use the same process to free yourself from the pain you have felt stuck in.

I had reached a threshold in my suffering. I had to gain an awareness of WHY I felt the way that I did. This is when I started peeling back the layers of my patterns of focus, my beliefs, and the things I was doing that were tearing me apart.

This awareness led me to the decision that I did not want to live that way any longer.

I had to choose not to live that story.

I had to really think about what I wanted most in life.

For me, that was freedom from my OCD. Freedom from my suffering.

I wanted to feel safe in my own skin. I wanted to know myself, love myself, and realize my own worth. I wanted to find purpose and something to live for.

I had to choose the story in life I DID want to live.

It was a story that would empower me to get what I wanted most in life.

It was a story that I would condition and role-play until that became the real me.

Would I believe that story right away? No. It would feel uncomfortable. Like I'm trying to convince myself of some mistruth.

But the discomfort in role-playing this new story of the person I wanted to be was much less painful than the discomfort of continuing to live the story that was slowly killing me.

This is what GOING FIRST is. It's DECIDING what story you want to live.

Condition it. Role-play it. Lean into the discomfort and awkwardness of that.

Become the person you need to become to live the life you dream of by acting as if you are already that person.

Think like them.

Act as they would.

Believe what that person would believe.

When I was twenty-three, I got a phone call from my father.

My father was my hero. He had never missed a single game of mine during my entire high school and college career. I loved making him proud. I looked up to him. His love meant so much to me.

He was crying when I answered the phone. Crying so hard that he couldn't speak.

I thought he was going to tell me he was sick or dying. My heart sank, and I waited in tortured anticipation for him to speak.

When he found his words, he said, "Someone told me you're gay. I couldn't possibly have a daughter that is GAY! I beg you, Siri, tell me this isn't true."

I froze, then shook from the inside out.

"Dad, it's true. I'm gay. But I am the same me. Please, just love me anyway."

He hung up the phone. I had just exposed the most vulnerable part of myself and was completely rejected. My heart broke into a million pieces.

I didn't hear from him for the next two years. Nothing.

After that, I was lucky to get a phone call on Christmas.

His rejection ripped me to pieces. It made me feel like all that I had achieved, all that I had become, meant absolutely NOTHING now that I was gay.

Being gay was so wrong, so shameful, that it could rip a lifetime of my father's love out of my hands in an instant.

When this happened, I had two choices.

1. Live the story that he was telling me: That being gay means I am worthless. I should be ashamed. I will be rejected and will never be able to find success or love in this world. His rejection told me I was not love-able, by myself or by another.

2. I am gay. Living authentically in my truth is where all my power lies. Being me is what matters most! If I live life bringing all of who I am into it, I will be able to tap into my fullest potential and be all that I am meant to be in this lifetime.

I was NOT willing to live the story he was telling me. Brokenhearted and filled with angst, I had to find all my strength within to decide what story I DID want to live. Even if I didn't believe it in that moment, I would find a way to become the person that did!

At twenty-three years old, feeling lost after losing my dad's love, I discovered triathlon.

I went and watched a friend of mine racing in a triathlon. I was in awe of the diversity I witnessed and the extraordinary heart and soul people were putting into this challenge they had chosen.

There were people of all ages, sizes, and ability levels. They were pushing themselves, it seemed, beyond what they thought they were capable of. It was this glorious personal challenge, unique to each participant. Everyone was coming up against their own limiting beliefs and embracing the invitation to find more, become more, and do something they had never done before.

THIS would be the vehicle through which I would find love and respect for myself. This would be how I could find out what I am really made of. I would build respect for myself and strengthen from the inside out so that one day I could live that life that I dreamed of.

The only problem? I was twenty-three years old and didn't know how to swim!

Many would question why I would do something I had no background in.

Isn't that what truly living is all about? As Eleanor Roosevelt said, "You must do the thing you think you cannot do."

I quickly convinced my friend, Lynn, to teach me how to swim, properly ride a bike, and how to run over a long distance rather than sprinting after a puck or ball.

I did my first race a few months later, finishing dead last.

I had never felt so ALIVE in my entire life.

On that day, I decided I wanted to be the best in the world in the sport one day.

I could have told myself the story that I don't know how to swim, and as cool as this sport looked and no matter how pulled I was to do it, this sport wasn't for me.

But I was not willing to live that story!

I had a deep, emotional reason WHY I had to achieve this goal.

I was on a desperate mission to prove to myself, most importantly, that even as a gay woman I could achieve something spectacular. I could inspire others. I could make a difference in this world, and I could be loved by another, and even more importantly, love myself.

I needed to do this for me!

So, instead of living the old story that would have prevented me from even trying, I wrote a new story:

I am a great athlete. I know how to work hard. I feel this insatiable passion and hunger to take on this goal, and one day, I will become a triathlon world champion.

Changing my story led to me doing what that "future me," the one that could win a world championship, would do in every moment.

Even though I sucked at first, I found a coach and immersed myself in the sport.

I modeled the very best athletes in the world.

I lived every day as if I was that person that would be a champion one day.

With laser focus and unwavering discipline, I was doing what needed to be done every day to become the person I needed to become to eventually win a world championship.

Later, as a high-performance triathlon coach, I had one athlete that wanted to become an Ironman world champion.

My first thought was "I have never raced an Ironman. I have only ever done Olympic distance triathlons (a two-hour race, as opposed to the nine-plus hours required for an

Ironman). How could I ever coach this great athlete to a crown in a sport I had no experience in?"

But I WANTED to be that person to coach her toward that goal. So, I had to re-narrate that story.

I told myself, "I went from not being able to swim to becoming a world champion eight years later. I have grit, experience, heart, and expertise in winning championships, and I will coach my athletes to world championship crowns."

What would that person do? What would that person believe?

She would learn all about Ironman and stack her proof of why she had everything she needed to guide her athlete to achieving this goal.

Role-play the new story. Condition the new story. You will then become THAT person.

In 2019, I was diagnosed with acute myeloid leukemia intensified by a genetic mutation that was going to make it very difficult to treat, much less survive.

I could have listened to the statistics that said it was the end.

I was NOT willing to live that story!

I went first in deciding what story I wanted to live.

I am going to survive, and I am going to THRIVE.

Did I believe that in that moment? No! I was terrified. I was in shock. I was devastated, but if I didn't change the meaning of what was happening to me, I would not be here today.

If I didn't change the story to empower me, I would have ended up being just another statistic.

You can see the power of changing your story.

Change your story. Change your life!

Here are a few brief examples in my life, and I hope you will think of the same in your own life:

I wanted to speak on Tony Robbins's stage even though I had never spoken in front of a crowd.

But sometimes what one needs to say is too important to let fear get in the way! My first event was the Tony Robbins Leadership Academy in Coronado Bay, CA in 2017.

I wanted to rescue and ban the slaughter of American horses for human consumption even though I only had one year of experience with these beautiful animals and knew nothing about lobbying to pass a bill.

I became the person that could do this, rescuing 194 horses from the slaughter pipeline with our 501(c)(3), Believe Ranch and Rescue, and then raising awareness about the brutal practice significantly through our 501(c)(4), Horses in Our Hands.

Through our lobbying and education, we decreased the total amount of horses being slaughtered from sixty thousand per year to twenty-six thousand.

We have reached eighty-four million homes through our awareness campaign and have sent 207,000 letters to legislators asking them to pass the Save America's Forgotten Equines (SAFE) Act, which would ban horse slaughter for good.

All these things required me to give up my old stories that would have prevented me from even trying.

What stories have you been telling yourself that have prevented you from acting on something that you're passionate about? What stories have you been telling yourself that have kept you from having the deep, loving relationships you yearn for or the success that you strive for?

I needed to rewrite those stories to become the person who could achieve all that I wanted to achieve.

Just like me, you will be faced with defining moments where how you respond to that moment will determine the entire trajectory of your life. When standing at those inevitable intersections in life you must decide what story you want to live.

You alone get to decide what to make of a great challenge you are faced with. You alone get to decide what painful rejection will mean to you.

The meaning we give the things that happen to us has an undeniable effect on the directions our lives take.

You alone get to decide what is possible for you.

It's time for me to guide you on how to change your stories so that you can live in alignment with what you want and what matters most to you.

First, you must recognize the stories that are holding you back.

One thing you must know is that our stories are software, not hardware. They can be updated, changed, removed, and replaced.

Remember:

- You get to GO FIRST in deciding what story you want to live.

- Our stories are software, not hardware. They can be updated, changed, removed, and replaced.

- The meaning we give the things that happen to us has an undeniable effect on the directions our lives take. Reframe and find an empowering meaning.

ASSIGNMENT: CHANGE YOUR STORY, CHANGE YOUR LIFE

Take some time to answer the following questions to become aware of the stories that you are living.

What do you want most in life?

What is getting in the way of you having that?

What is your current story?

When thinking about your current story, let these questions guide you:

What do you believe about it?
What do you feel about it?
What does it mean to you?
What is missing or lacking?
What do you believe it SHOULD be?

What parts of your story cause you the most concern and grief?

Which part of your story causes the most disruption in your life?

What are they disrupting? Describe in detail:

Which of these stories creates the most misalignment with your values?

Does this story take you where you want to go in life?

If the answer is NO, what story do you tell yourself to justify it? (Especially considering the thousands of hours it consumes.)

TIME TO WRITE YOUR NEW STORY

In doing this, think about the opposite of the story you have now.

Write the opposite of each part of your story here:

In crafting your new story, don't think small, think BIG!! The following questions can help guide you.

What do you believe about work, relationships, or health in your new story?
Who are you?
What do you believe?
What do you feel?
What do you KNOW?
What does it mean to you?
What do you experience?
How do you show up?

Write your new story in detail.

ROLE-PLAY this NEW STORY in every way possible.

In this situation, what would the "future me" do, think, focus on, believe, or feel?

Shift to doing what the future you would do.

You must condition this.

At first, it will feel awkward and hard. STICK TO IT!

Just like learning how to swim, it will feel hard at first, but the more you practice, the more natural it feels. Be consistent! Be focused and COMMIT!!!

It's up to you to do that.

You don't just write the new story, and it happens. You must condition the new story. Role-play it until it becomes you.

Ask yourself in every moment, "What would the 'future me' believe in this moment? What would the 'future me' do in this moment?"

You must lean in.

Put habits and rituals in place that will help you condition the new story.

What are three things you can do every day to help you condition your new story?

One small recommendation: read your new story every day!

Chapter 4

THE POWER OF IDENTITY AND AUTHENTICITY

*W*ho you believe you are will determine what you can do in your life.

There is a difference between believing and knowing.

Oftentimes, our identity was created before we even had a choice to decide on our own.

Sam is so sensitive. Cat struggles. Mackenzie has a hard time dealing with conflict. Petra is an amazing problem solver. Lou is delicate or strong. The list goes on.

Our parents, teachers, siblings, friends, and even us now love to label people so we can better understand them and anticipate what they need or desire.

Society also tells us as we are growing up who we should be, what we shouldn't do, how we should live our lives, what we should find important, and how we should act in certain situations.

Eager to please, many of us do all those things we SHOULD do. It leads us to become someone that fits in but feels like a stranger in their own skin.

Can you relate to this?

In college, battling my obsessive-compulsive disorder, all my fear was wrapped up in losing my family: them dying or getting sick and me dying or getting sick.

They formed my identity. I was my mom's protector. I was the source of my dad's pride and joy. I was "doing" everything I needed to do to be a good daughter. I was loving, kind, giving, achieving, excelling, hardworking, and never a problem.

I discovered the formula for making my parents happy and proud. So, that is who I would be.

Going off to college, I could no longer protect my mom. (Even though she didn't need protecting. That was the story I made up and believed due to my fear.)

I would see my dad a couple times a week when he would come to watch a game of field hockey, ice hockey, or lacrosse.

He came to see me perform. Would I succeed or would I fail in making him proud?

It was all about that, not about me.

The pressure was so heavy. Again, it was pressure I put on myself. He was there because he was happy to see me and to enjoy watching his daughter play sports.

My identity was the achiever—the sports star, the good girl, the strong girl.

Everything I did would be measured by whether I was all those things on any given day.

When I reached the peak of my OCD, it manifested as total exhaustion.

I couldn't continue to show up, put on a brave face, perform, and achieve. I was just so tired.

I needed relief. I was the hamster running nonstop on the wheel, unable to get off.

It was miraculously at this time I became aware of Tony Robbins. This incredible man was so young but had such deep wisdom. Where did he get it from? How did he know all these things that I needed?

The most powerful epiphany I had was that only I could get myself off this hamster wheel. It was all up to me!

All the discipline I brought to my classes, my studies, my practices, and my games I needed to redirect to my focus. I had to shift focus to what I wanted, not what I feared.

I had to give things a different meaning.

For example: When my mom got divorced, I told myself she was devasted, broken, and so vulnerable. She needed me to keep her alive.

I changed the meaning to…

When my mom got divorced, she finally found FREEDOM. She now had the freedom to live in a way that brought out the best in her and inspired her. She could now have all the things she was unable to have while being the arm candy to her man. She could now be all that she was destined to be.

It was kind of like how I felt right in that moment at Brown University. I finally understood that it was all up to me. I felt this freedom—this sense of purpose. I felt in control for the first time in a decade.

One of the first things I needed to do to continue this path was to figure out who I was.

I really didn't know.

I decided to sign up for summer work at Club Med as a G.O. (gentil organisateur).

Years back, my mom had taken my sister and me to a Club Med in Haiti.

I loved it because you could choose from several different activities to partake in every day: windsurfing, snorkeling, water aerobics, bocce ball, volleyball, etc.

What I didn't like was that everyone wanted to talk to you. They would pull you out of your beach chair to get you to do a water aerobics class or join a volleyball game.

I wanted it to be my choice. I needed to deliberate on whether it was the right time or the right thing for me to do. That answer would come from analyzing what my mom needed and if it looked like she was all set, I would do it.

Anyhow, here I was filling out an application for Club Med in Huatulco, Mexico.

They asked whether I was fluent in another language.

I had taken ten years of French but really could not have a conversation. But I checked the box. YES! French.

Then they had some questions about personality. Are you introverted? Or extroverted?

Extroverted. CHECK!

That was not the case. But what if it was? What if I was at my core extroverted but my identity required me to be introverted?

Off I went. I decided on the airplane that since no one would know who I am, I could show up as whomever I wanted.

They wouldn't know the difference.

So, I arrived happy, excited, confident, friendly, talkative, and eager to inspire.

This was who I wanted to be.

I was going to try this on for size and see if it fit.

It felt very strange but also so liberating, trying on all these different characteristics. Some felt nothing like me, some just felt so good. It showed me that this was something I had left unexpressed until this moment. But it was a part of me that felt enlightened.

Every day I would run around convincing vacationers WHY they should take my water aerobics class. It would energize them and allow them to enjoy the tremendous buffet with no guilt. I would make them laugh. I would make them smile. The more I did this, the more I felt happier. I felt more relaxed. I felt more like myself.

I would teach three classes a day. Everyone who had been working there for a long time said they couldn't believe my ability to get so many vacationers to join the classes. Usually there would only be a handful of people participating. My classes never had less than fifteen people.

For the first time in my life, I realized I could be a leader. I could inspire people. I could encourage people to do things differently that would truly benefit them.

My goal at Club Med was to help make the best vacation for these people that had probably been dreaming of this trip for a long time. I wanted to bring out the best in them—have them do things that I knew would help them to feel more energized, happy, confident, and fulfilled.

I was there for a full month. There were no TVs and no way to call home.

This was the first time I was literally on my own, without contact with my mom, dad, or family.

On my way there, this terrified me, but I had learned not to obsess over thoughts that made me feel bad and could potentially prevent me from taking this opportunity. So, instead, I focused on what an incredible opportunity this would be to find myself. I was going to discover parts of myself that I had not allowed myself to explore.

I was stuck in the identity that was only bringing me pain.

I needed to find myself, and this separation would allow that to happen.

When I got home, mom was alive and well. She was playing lots of tennis with her friends, teaching aerobics classes, and loving life. My dad still loved me even though I wasn't out breaking records or achieving goals on a sports field. This reassured me that what I had told myself for so long about who I needed to be to maintain the love of my parents was a load of BS.

I came back knowing that I was a leader. I had a sense of humor. I loved bringing sunshine into people's lives. When I was confident, I had so much more to give. When I opened the shades, rolled down the windows, and breathed in all that was me, I became alive.

I returned to Brown that fall with a newfound confidence and a willingness to explore and try new things. I brought excitement to deepen my relationship with myself.

Part of this exploration process was letting myself do things that weren't necessarily supported by others. I wasn't holding myself back because of what other people thought I SHOULD do, but I followed my heart and did what I felt I MUST.

I had been recruited to Brown University as an ice hockey player.

It was my favorite sport. It's a beautiful mix of endurance, grit, skill, finesse, and strength.

When I got to Brown, I also wanted to play field hockey and lacrosse. There was one coach for both teams. She gave me an ultimatum. Do both field hockey and lacrosse or just ice hockey, but you can't do all three.

This broke my heart. I was going to have to give up my favorite sport.

With my anxiety at an all-time high, I knew how important it was for me to keep busy and focused through sport. If I only played ice hockey, then that would leave many months where I would not have the therapeutic benefits of being focused on a sport.

Although I loved playing field hockey and lacrosse, a part of me felt that I had really let myself down by not allowing myself to do all three. There is always a way.

When I returned to school from Club Med my senior year, I decided that I would no longer be and do what everyone else wanted me to do. I went into my coach's office and said, "I am going to play ice hockey this year." She looked at me, cheeks flushed red with anger, and responded, "NO, you will NOT."

I explained that this was what I was recruited for and that I would never forgive myself if I didn't at least play one year.

She replied, "You do that, and I will do everything in my power to keep you on the bench. You will never play a game for me."

I could not believe her unwillingness to let me explore what I was capable of.

In my anger, I found this unbridled confidence that blew out of my mouth. "I will make it impossible for you NOT to play me."

This lit a fire inside of me that I would work harder and smarter than ever before. I would be so prepared and so crucial to the team that she simply could not keep me on the bench.

For the first time in my life, I was standing up for myself.

I was going to be the first female athlete in Brown's history to play three varsity sports in the same year.

I didn't realize that until just recently.

No one gets to tell you what is possible or not possible for you.

Only you get to decide that. Only you get to decide what you are capable of.

What was born on that day is a part of my identity that I believe is one of my greatest strengths: believing in all possibilities.

I was willing to be the FIRST.

How can you ever know what you are truly capable of if you are not trying to do what you don't think you can do, every day?

Don't tell me something is impossible.

That will give me even more reason to TRY.

Every great invention started with someone believing in something that no one had ever seen before. They never gave up until it was created.

YOU are the creator of your life. Think Big. Dream Big. Reach for the moon and the worst that can happen is that you will land among the stars.

I AM GAY.

I AM STRAIGHT.

Does it matter? Does this really have to define who you are as a human being?

Don't squash all of who you are into a tiny label that is only one part of you.

Who else are you?

Are you kind and loving? Hard-working and committed?

Do you have a great sense of humor? Are you a philanthropist? Do you love helping others?

You are so much more than your career—so much more than your sexual orientation, your political party, or the size of your bank account.

When my dad called me on that dreadful day, he was shocked at the truth that I was gay. The first thing I said to him was "Dad, I am the same me."

This wasn't enough.

He hung up the phone with an exclamation point, proclaiming that who I am was not okay.

I spoke in earlier chapters about the story I had to choose to live from that day forward.

I was given two choices: Believe what he was telling me. That because I am gay, I am worthless. I am an embarrassment. I am a sinner. I will only experience pain and I will never find love.

Or choose the story that was the truth.

I am gay. I know who I am, and this gives me a centeredness that will allow me to put all my energy into creating the life of my dreams. Being gay will be my superpower because that is my authentic self. Living authentically will allow me to be all that I can be in this life, as all energy will be with me and not spent trying to be something I am not.

"I know who I am, and this gives me a centeredness that will allow me to put all my energy into creating the life of my dreams."

As hard as it was to not do everything in my power to not lose my father, that decision would have made for a lifetime of pain and suffering.

Short-term devastating pain and grief from my loss would ultimately lead to a much more comfortable future: not having to pretend, not having to hide, and not having to constantly show up as others required. I would just show up as me.

Living authentically gave me a sense of peace within my own body. A peace that had eluded me for so many years. The decision I made to be me gave me a sense of confidence knowing that I had my own support, my own blessing. That was enough, for now.

I started triathlon soon after that call with my father.

Triathlon would be the vehicle through which I would find myself, find respect for myself, find worthiness from within, and hopefully and most importantly, find love for myself.

If I was going to live every second of every day, every week, every month, every year, every decade with me and only me, I really wanted to like myself, trust myself, and respect myself.

I chose myself and vowed to stay true to myself forever more.

That didn't happen.

Six years into my triathlon career, I got offered an unbelievable sponsorship from a high-profile company.

I hadn't even won anything yet. I was, at best, average in this sport. But they offered me the moon (for triathlon standards). They probably didn't think I would get the results that would bring me the biggest bonuses. But I felt that with their support I could finally stop working sixty hours a week while trying to train as a professional athlete and that would give me the chance to really make progress.

When I went into their New York offices to sign the deal, they had one last "deal breaker":

Grow your hair long.

Get yourself a boyfriend.

"This is a family-oriented company. You have to fit the bill here, otherwise we can't move forward."

I had to choose between myself or this deal that could be exactly what I needed to finally get to the level I dreamed of in the sport.

I signed the agreement. I left the room, walked straight back into my closet, and slammed the door shut behind me.

I abandoned myself. It was so painful. I felt so shallow. I felt so ashamed.

I understand in hindsight why I took that deal. It was giving me the opportunity to remove all financial stress and put all my energy into achieving my goal of becoming a world champion.

I must forgive myself for this. I did the best that I could with what I knew at the time.

And at the time, this felt like the best decision for me.

I left NYC and didn't get a haircut for another six months. I got a boyfriend, and I had an amazing sponsor. My future in the sport looked bright, but my respect and trust in myself took a huge hit. Ashamed of the decision I had made, I had a hard time believing that I deserved anything good to happen in my career.

By allowing this group to convince me to change who I am in a ten-minute conversation, I felt so weak. Pathetic.

My only response to this judgment that ate me from the inside out was to train harder than ever before. I had to dig deeper than ever before and prove my strength to myself that way.

Everything came from an energy of force. I had to prove to myself I was strong, not weak. I had to prove to my dad that even as a gay woman I could achieve great things. I could inspire others and make a difference in this world.

After winning the world championship in 2001, I vowed I would NEVER abandon myself again. I would never put myself in a position again where I would shun every part of what makes me, me.

When we live an identity that isn't true to us, we feel unhappy. Incongruent.

We must fight the feelings of pretense and shame by DOING.

Yes, you can achieve great things in this state, but at what cost to your heart and soul?

You don't have to be what you were, or what your parents were, or what someone else thinks you are. All you need to be is yourself.

Don't know who that is? Let me ask you these questions:

What makes you feel most alive?

What drains you?

What are your top values? The things that matter most to you and drive you in your life?

(You did this exercise in part 1.)

Your identity will change over time, like retiring from a certain profession, for example.

My wife retired from racing professionally in triathlon in 2017. She had one of the most brilliant careers, breaking the world Iron-distance record along with Chrissie Wellington at Challenge Roth in 2009 and having won six Iron-distance triathlons. She was also a two-time Junior World champion. For twenty years triathlon was her life, she was a triathlete. That was her identity.

Why is it so hard for many professional triathletes to end their careers?

Because it is all they know. They live and breathe triathlon and all their worth lies in this sport they have committed their lives to.

My wife for twenty-plus years would get up each day with one goal in mind: training herself to be the fastest, fittest, and strongest triathlete she could be.

The target was to win races.

Her identity was wrapped tightly up in triathlon.

This is how we met.

I was coaching her and was holding a camp in Noosa, Australia.

As a coach, I had sharp boundaries with my athletes. I am the coach; they are the athlete. We didn't fraternize.

One of my athletes who organized this training camp came to pick me up at the airport. She said, "This camp is going to be amazing. The only problem is that you must share a house with one of your athletes."

I replied, "I would rather sleep in a tent on the street than share a house with an athlete."

She asked me to just look at the house, so I could see for myself the space and if it could possibly work.

Who was the athlete I would be sharing with?

"Rebekah Keat," she said.

Somehow that made it a little bit more all right.

She showed me this gorgeous house on the beach. A famous Australian actor had offered his place as he was a triathlete and was thrilled to help us out.

I walked inside and saw that I would have the upstairs, and Bek would have the downstairs. The only thing we would have to share was the kitchen.

Every night, I would eat before Bek and leave before she started cooking her own dinner.

But eventually, I would linger a bit longer after my meal, or she would come in a bit earlier. We started getting to know each other better just as people. We had so much in common: a love for our animals, a love for family, and an appreciation for life.

She made me laugh deep-belly laughs, and she sparked something inside of me that made me come alive.

We fell in love, and the rest is history.

Bek had achieved so much in her long career. She was one of the greatest female Iron-distance athletes in the history of the sport. I could tell she was getting tired. She was getting injured more often and just didn't seem to love it anymore.

In 2016, Tony Robbins and his wife Sage invited Bek and me to come to an Unleash the Power Within (UPW) event in San Jose, CA.

I was beside myself excited.

I was just on Tony Robbins's podcast, and we had the most amazing talk. I was able to thank him for being my greatest mentor for the last twenty years and share just how his teachings had impacted my life.

That podcast ended up being one of his top-downloaded podcasts—over three million downloads.

I couldn't believe it!

Originally, when they asked me to be on the show, I thought they wanted one of my superstar athletes that I was coaching. I sent them their email addresses. They responded by saying that it was me they wanted—what a privilege and what a gift.

This moment led to the change in direction that put me squarely on the path of my mission and purpose.

I begged Bek to come with me to San Jose. She said she couldn't imagine anything worse than jumping up and down like a crazy person for fourteen hours a day. She was NOT interested.

I began to worry a lot about our relationship.

I was on the verge of this period of intense learning and growth, eager to become more and expand my impact on many more lives than just my athletes.

This was a dream opportunity to learn from my greatest mentor by walking the path of his every seminar to acquire more tools and a greater understanding of myself. This would allow me to truly live my life to my highest potential.

Finally, she said yes. I told her she could spend most of the day training and just join me when she was done.

The first day she trained most of the day but came for the last few hours.

The next day, intrigued, she came for half the day.

On the third day out of four, she didn't miss a single second.

She woke up to the undisputable truth that she was so much more than just a triathlete.

At UPW, she dug deep into all aspects of who she was as a human being: an advocate for animals and human rights, a giver, and a bright and inspiring leader.

She began to explore all the other things in life she would want to do.

Before this event, the idea of not having triathlon scared her.

What would she do? Who would she be? The emptiness that that thinking brought her was intolerable. She would then go into periods of deep stress as her body was breaking down and the end seemed imminent.

But now she had tools. They were the tools to navigate from racing to retirement and retirement to the next chapter in her life.

She knew she had to be gentle with herself as it would be the first major identity shift she would ever go through.

This was the end of one chapter and the beginning of a new one. She could create whatever she dreamed of.

She asked herself the key questions that I want to share with you:

Who are you going to be now?

What lights you up?

What will you create?

How will you add value to other people?

She would hold herself to the same standards she had as an athlete but in these different areas.

Identity should be tied to who you are, not what you do.

Retiring athletes need a restart, a pivot.

All those years that Bek had spent training to be the best in triathlon had also strengthened character traits that would be the ingredients for all future successes in whatever lit her up: resilience, discipline, work ethic, passion, focus, and desire.

She came with me to every Tony Robbins seminar.

She wrapped her arms around every event and soaked it all up.

Together we traveled this tremendous path of growth that united us more deeply and set Bek on her future career path at lightning speed.

Since 2017, Bek has created two businesses with me: the Team Sirius Tri Club (www.teamsiriustriclub.com) and the Sirius Squad (www.siriussquad.com).

Together, we have also created two nonprofits, rescuing horses from slaughter and banning horse slaughter altogether.

She has taken course after course, learning all about social media targeting and influence.

She takes all our projects to the next level with her incredible talents in this area.

She didn't know she had the ability to do all these things, but she told herself the story she could and then she went about becoming that person that WOULD!

She has deeply impacted so many lives, giving her a fulfillment that was unmatched by triathlon.

She has blossomed into this multi-dimensional powerhouse of a human being. She is beautiful, giving, inspiring, and making amazing things happen in the world.

YOU too can make a change like this. It is all in your hands.

Are you living life in alignment with what matters most?

In the assignment that follows, you will audit your life and will be able to answer that question.

If you are not in alignment, that would explain why you are unhappy or dissatisfied in certain aspects of it.

If you are happy in certain aspects of your life, this would show that you are living true to yourself in that area.

So, you can see that uncovering your top values becomes a moral GPS. It gives you the knowledge you need to make the right decisions for you. These are decisions about what career to pursue, who to share your life with, or how to fill your free time.

Knowing who you are and what you really want will help you choose a path that will take you where you want to go.

I truly believe that you can have everything in life. But to do that you must

1. know who you are;
2. know what you want; and
3. make decisions that are congruent with those things.

Be you. Bring all of you into this game of life. Yes, this takes courage, but what you will find is that you will be firing on all cylinders and thus tapping into your fullest potential, finding a way to all that you want in life.

BEING is where it is at.

Being YOU. ALL of who you are.

Don't leave any part of who you are on the bench.

If you do, you will show up less than your best.

It will deny you the depth of relationship you desire and the impact you can have on the world.

Remember:

- Don't hold yourself back because of what others think you should do, instead, follow your heart and do what you feel you must.

- To find joy and fulfillment, live life in alignment with what matters most to you.

- BE YOU! Don't leave any part of who you are on the bench.

- Living fearlessly and authentically will enable you to live to your highest potential.

ASSIGNMENT: IDENTITY WORKSHEET

Let's take time now to figure out who you really are.

Time to move past the stories people told you about who you are.

What parts of your identity were never yours in the first place?

What parts of who you are were placed upon you by society, parents, or yourself while you were just trying to fit in?

Often, your identity has so many layers that you lose sight of the real you.

Let's peel off the layers of your identity that weren't yours in the first place. It's time to reveal your true self. Underneath it all. Your angel within, in all its glory.

From this exercise, you will better understand the people and things that have shaped your behaviors and decisions and thus, how you live your life.

The parts of your identity that aren't the real you get in the way of living your best life.

Influences that can shape our identity are our parents, siblings, friends, teachers, social media, the media we watch, and our education.

I remember my parents always saying "Siri is so shy" when I was a little kid. This became my identity. But was it really me? No, I just became that because that was what I was constantly told.

Your assignment:

Part 1: Shaping forces, growing up

Things my parents and loved ones have said about me:

1.

2.

3.

Who did I need to be so my parents are pleased or I will feel loved?

Is that who I really am?

Who did I need to be for my friends to accept me?

How was I required to act to make my parents, teachers, and friends happy?

Do I still follow these same rules?

Does it feel authentic to me?

The two to three people, events, or things that have shaped my identity:

Briefly describe:

1.

2.

3.

The three times in my life where I felt totally grounded in who I was and what I was doing—the times where I felt genuinely happy and fulfilled.

Who was with me? What was I focused on? What was I doing every day? What emotions did I feel most of the time? What was missing?

1.

2.

3.

The three times in my life where I was unhappy, unfulfilled, or disappointed.

What was I doing? Who was I with? What was I focused on? What emotions did I feel most of the time? What was missing?

1.

2.

3.

Present Identity:

Who am I?

What are my greatest qualities?

If I asked those closest to me what my strongest qualities are, they would say:

I am most proud of:

1.

2.

3.

What makes me feel most alive? Energized? Inspired?

1.

2.

3.

What matters most to you?

1.

2.

3

What brings out the best in me?

What brings out the worst in me?

What area of my life am I happiest with? Why? What makes it so good?

What area of my life am I unhappy with? Why? What makes it disappointing or hard?

The best way to find your true self is to focus on what matters most to you.

What are my top five values?

1.

2.

3.

4.

5.

Am I living life in alignment with those top values? At work? In relationships? With my health? Within myself?

Am I compromising my values for another?

Do I have clear boundaries in relationships, in work, and with myself?

What would it look like to live fearlessly authentic in every aspect of my life?

Who am I?

Who am I not?

What actions can I take today to start living my life more authentically?

    1.

    2.

    3.

Chapter 5

THE POWER OF COURAGE

Being afraid but doing it anyway—that is courage. Courage is required on this journey and that is why it is one of the key stops along the Power Line.

Courage gets us to walk through the fire, trusting in ourselves and in our ability to weather the flames.

Fear is always with us.

When I was in college, my fear manifested as OCD. When I was diagnosed with leukemia, one of my biggest fears was that my wife would no longer love me. Another fear was having people see me suffer. I had this belief that I could not show my suffering as it went against who I was as a human being. I choose to be happy, hopeful, and NOT to suffer.

I had to come to terms with the fact that I was going to suffer and that I needed to love and accept myself through those moments.

What would I say to someone I love the most if they were going through something similar?

Would I say, "Come on, be happy. Don't suffer. Get your shit together," or would I say, "I know this time is tough. Be patient. Be brave. And know that this too shall pass. Focus as much as you can on how good it will feel to be healthy and strong again. But, for now, know that you are so loved. I am here for you. I will not leave your side, and I know that you are going to get through this."

These are the words I needed to speak to myself. I needed to have compassion, love, and patience for myself. It is through this time that I truly realized just how important self-love is.

Self-love is loving yourself, speaking to yourself, and believing in yourself in every moment as you would your most beloved.

So how do you manage fear? My belief is that we must accept that fear is natural and oftentimes a great motivator.

For example, when racing as a professional triathlete, I would feel overwhelming fear before the start of every race. Rather than letting this debilitate me, I had to give this fear another meaning. I decided to look at how this fear was serving me.

When fearful, it put me in a place where I became laser-focused on doing what I needed to do to perform to the best of my ability.

Fear mobilized everything I needed inside of me to perform the way I wanted to.

Think about dealing with a scary situation, like a child choking and the fear it strikes within you. But it leads you to take swift, focused action to come to the child's rescue.

So, what if we saw fear as our friend? As an ally?

Fear can hold us back, but it can also push us to do great things. It is through our fear that we learn and grow. It is through fear that we strengthen ourselves as we tap into all the courage within. When we learn to use our fear, it can serve us. Fear directs us, filling us with adrenaline that focuses our attention and drives us to new heights.

Be afraid, but do it anyway. You can build the courage muscle by doing something every day to push past what you fear.

This requires emotional resilience.

I know this well.

I forged this superpower in the fires of training to become a World Triathlon champion.

This superpower ultimately led to my most beautiful triumph, surviving AML.

I will always remember my first week of training with Brett in Switzerland.

He kept telling me to go harder, and I said, "I can't go any harder than I am right now."

That is what it felt like. But was it true? Did I have more in me but was just too afraid to see what that would feel like?

Every day, running on the treadmill, I would just put the speed faster than what I believed I could do. On the first day, just thirty seconds at that speed seemed impossible.

It hurt so bad, but I survived.

The next day, one minute at that speed.

It hurt bad, but I survived.

The next day ninety seconds, etc.

Eventually, I was running 10 km at that pace, which at one point seemed impossible.

I built up my resistance to the discomfort of going beyond what I thought I could.

This was a necessary step in becoming the athlete I needed to be to win a world championship.

Take little steps each day to get out of your comfort zone. Leaning INTO the fear will bring you one step closer to not only putting out the flames of that specific fear but to becoming who you dream of becoming.

So, here is your task:

1. Do something every day that scares you.
2. Make it a little scarier each day.
3. Document your progress and celebrate your courage.

How can you ever know what you are truly capable of if you are not trying to do what you don't think you can, every day? You must get out of your comfort zone.

You are so much more powerful and capable than you could ever imagine.

Remember this:

- Build your courage muscle: do something that scares you every day!

- Fear can hold us back, but it can also push us to do great things. It is through our fear that we learn and grow. It is through fear that we strengthen ourselves as we tap into all the courage within. When we learn to use our fear, it can serve us. Fear directs us, filling us with adrenaline that focuses our attention and drives us to new heights.

- Be afraid, but do it anyway. This is courage.

ASSIGNMENT: OVERCOMING FEAR

Day 1:

What can I do today that scares me? Don't overthink it, just go do it!

Write down how it went. Did you survive? How did you feel? Celebrate your courage!

Day 2:

What can I do today that is a little bit scarier? A bit more uncomfortable?

How did it go? What happened? How did you feel? Celebrate your courage!

Day 3:

What can I do today that is a bit scarier than yesterday?

How did it go? What did you do? How did you feel? Celebrate your courage!

Continue this for the next week. Say yes to doing things that take you out of your comfort zone every day.

How can you ever know what you are truly capable of if you are not trying to do what you don't think you can? You must get out of your comfort zone.

Chapter 6

THE POWER
OF GRATITUDE

The year 2000:

I spent ten months on a mission to make the USA Olympic team for the 2000 Summer Olympic Games in Sydney.

I decided that to find my greatest strength, I needed to do this on my own, inspired by great athletes like Mark Allen and Brad Bevan. Those lone soldiers had a laser focus and an internal drive fueling their everyday quest to be the very best.

So, I left the USA and flew out to Cronulla, Australia. I got a nine-month lease on a little third-floor apartment near the beach.

I had a small sofa, a small, round, one-person dining table, an altitude tent for my bed, and a whole army of cockroaches.

I laid out a plan with my coach to diligently go about checking off all the necessary boxes of training tasks and mental exercises so that I could arrive on the Sydney Olympic qualifying race day one million percent prepared.

Every single day, I trained meticulously. I followed each hard training session with proper fueling, recovery, and reflection.

I was eating dinner by 5:00 every night, doing my abdominal routine by 7:15, and in bed by 8:00 every day like clockwork. Before I went to sleep, I went through my "perfect race" from start to finish, every single night for nine months.

I visualized every aspect of the course from my arrival on site, to my set up of transition, to my warmup, to the first dive into the Sydney harbor.

My visualization saw me executing to perfection the necessary plan to secure my spot on the US Olympic team.

As I stood on the pontoon on April 16, 2000, I had never felt so well prepared. I knew that I was in the form of my career thus far, and after a fourth-place finish on this same course a year earlier, I felt confident I could get the job done on this day.

The gun went off. We dove into the harbor with a clean dive and with exactly the start I had visualized for 365 nights in a row.

But then, about fifteen strokes in, I got an elbow to the head. As I ducked in reaction, the arm came up and around my shoulder, pushing me under the water, and I was subsequently swum over by the two people directly behind me.

I gasped for breath and tried to regain my composure, at which point the front pack had put about ten meters into me. I was now in the second pack.

I learned how to swim when I was twenty-three. Somehow, through relentless hard work and never-ending focus, I had improved my swim to the point of being able to hang on for dear life to the front pack if I got off to a smooth start. This, of course, was what I had been visualizing every night leading into this day's race.

So, what happened in that moment came as a total surprise to me, and because I had never prepared for ANYTHING BUT the perfect race, I was lost with how to manage this unforeseen circumstance.

I swam as hard as I could, more breathless than I should have been after the countless hard swims I had been doing in training.

I hung on for dear life as the second pack passed me, and the third pack came and dragged me along to the finish of the swim.

Once on the bike, again I was so unfamiliar with what was happening around me. None of the players I had imagined to be with me at this point of the race were with me. They were all minutes ahead. I got on my bike and pedaled my heart out, but not going anywhere—the pack I was with dropped me, and more and more people kept flying by me like I was standing still.

I was racing as if I had never trained before in my life.

I was frozen.

I was detached.

I was distraught.

I was choking.

I lost control over my emotions and my mind, and I quit. The most important race of my career thus far.

I felt like a complete failure.

I had proven my biggest fear that I would never be enough.

I wanted to climb into a hole and never come out. Shame buried me, not offering a crack of light to see any hope for my future.

The beauty of life is that no matter what is going on in your experience, the sun will always rise again.

My mind began transporting me back to those moments in college where I couldn't bear the thought of another moment being me.

What had I done then? How did I survive that time that felt so hopeless?

I had to participate in my own rescue. Right now.

I knew what to do. I had done it back then, and I would do it again now. I MUST.

All night I had been driving myself into deeper depression thinking about how far I had to go. I was thinking about everything I was missing that I needed to achieve my dream. I was thinking about my competitors that were moving forward as I swiftly fell backward. I was thinking about everything that was wrong and fearing everything that could go wrong in the future.

I had to remind myself of the mantra that had gotten me to where I was on this day: I am either winning, or I am learning.

Why did that suddenly not come into frame today?

That was up to me to bring to the forefront of my mind.

It was up to me to reframe the whole situation. To shift my focus altogether.

From this space, I became present with what I could learn from what had transpired.

This led to a resourcefulness that led me to ask better questions.

What do I need to change?

How can I use this to become better?

I learned that expectations can destroy you.

I went into this race visualizing the perfect race every single night for 365 days.

The expectation was that because I had trained to my highest potential and visualized everything happening as it needed to that somehow it would all just fall into place.

WHAT A RECIPE FOR DISASTER.

My greatest mentor Tony Robbins has always said, "Trade your expectation for appreciation, and see your entire world change in an instant."

BOOM. That stopped me in my tracks.

Here I was lamenting the fact that I had failed so miserably, forgetting entirely JUST HOW FAR I had come!

Six years ago, I didn't even know how to swim!

Here I was, having competed at the OLYMPIC TRIALS!

WOW, I have come SO FAR!

Change the way you look at things and the things you look at will change.

Suddenly, I felt this extreme GRATITUDE and appreciation for how amazing it was that I had come so far in just six years. I saw my relentlessness, I saw my will, I saw my courage, I saw my determination, I saw my hunger and my resilience all at once and felt this overwhelming sense of complete and utter gratitude!

I reminded myself of WHY I took this goal on in the first place. I wanted to find an appreciation for myself. I wanted to prove to myself that I was worthy. That I could believe in myself. That I could back myself and create amazing things in my life. I wanted to prove to myself that I mattered, to ME!

Somewhere along the line, I lost touch with the real reasons why I was doing this and suddenly became obsessed with making the Olympic team, getting sponsors, winning prize money, and achieving world rankings.

This led to me approaching my training and racing inauthentically. It was in a way that did not positively inspire or move me to race to my fullest potential.

It was too much pressure. I wasn't doing it for the right reasons.

From this point forward, I decided that every day in training and in every single race I would go out with the intention of laying everything I had inside of me out on the racecourse. It was my way of showing my gratitude to GOD for having blessed me with this amazing resilience, toughness, relentlessness, spirit, courage, and energy to take on this impossible dream. I would express my gratitude and express my appreciation by putting my entire heart, soul, and spirit into every opportunity.

Racing with gratitude. Racing in appreciation. Racing was a celebration of all the hard work I had done and all that I was and who I was becoming in the process.

This liberated me. This freed me to truly tap into my fullest potential with an energy of flow, in alignment with everything that mattered most to me.

Often your greatest victory comes just two millimeters after your biggest, most profound defeat.

Why? Because that profound disappointment leads to an insatiable curiosity about why you failed so miserably. It leads you to explore what went wrong and what you could do differently. It leads you to pivot, change your approach, and reconnect to WHY you are doing this in the first place.

The massive growth and clarity that comes are often what you needed to take your performance to the next level.

Can you think back to one of your deepest struggles and see the gift that was revealed because of it?

My biggest defeat led to a beautiful reckoning with my soul. It was a reminder of who I am and what my purpose was. It forced me to focus on how far I had come rather than how far I had left to go. It led me to a space where I became fully present in everything in my life, and in me, which I was so deeply grateful for.

What can you appreciate about that disappointment in your life?

What did you learn from it? Who did you become because of it?

Gratitude is the bridge from despair to hope.

In March 2020, I was in the fight of my life. I had my bone marrow transplant on February 21.

This procedure was what we had hoped would save my life.

To prepare for this, Dr. Gutman had said that he first needed to wipe out my existing immune system to make room for the new one. It would take a massive bomb of chemo and radiation over a weeklong period. This was what it would take to give me the best chance of this working.

This process took me to just a shadow of my former self. But it did the trick.

As soon as my numbers were life-threateningly low, right before a complete shutdown of my system, I got my lifesaving transplant.

Clumps of hair dropped off my head and I felt as though I was shedding every part of who I was.

Was I going to just fade away? Was life as I knew it gone forever? Would I ever recover?

I remember lying in my hospital bed, every single machine imaginable attached to me.

So sick, so weak. I had lost twenty-five pounds and couldn't eat. I was so exhausted and terrified of what was going to happen next.

But I would catch myself, and I'd say, "Siri, this is not going to help you heal. This makes you feel worse. This makes you feel weaker."

So, I would change the channel. Change the channel to gratitude.

I would look over at my mom who had slept on the tiny couch in my room for thirty-plus nights.

I felt so grateful. I would think of my amazing wife who had never left my side, and I felt so grateful.

I would think of my sister and the umbilical cord donor that were giving me life. I felt so grateful.

I would think of the doctors and nurses who wanted me to win this fight almost as much as I did. I felt so grateful. I felt so grateful for the notes and prayers coming in from loved ones and strangers alike.

Gratitude was the bridge from despair to hope.

Gratitude gave me energy. Gratitude gave me hope.

Gratitude directed me down a different path that was necessary for me to find the strength I needed to win this fight.

Gratitude is always the answer.

Surviving this deadly disease gave me an incredible new appreciation for life.

I have always been a very grateful person, always finding the good in everything and appreciating the little things that can bring so much joy.

But this experience took that gratitude to a whole new level.

I became acutely aware of the gift of every single breath I took.

When I finally was able to start eating again, every bite felt like this beautiful gift. It was a gift I would cherish. I saw the life-giving benefits of whatever I put in my mouth. For so long, I couldn't eat at all. I missed those moments of sharing a wonderful meal with my wife and the connection we shared.

I missed the energy and satisfaction that comes after finishing a meal. I missed the opportunity to give my body what it needed to survive, thanking my body through the fuel I gave it.

The first breath of fresh air after leaving the hospital where I had been indoors for over a month felt like the most beautiful elixir, filling my lungs with freedom, life, and energy.

Holding my dogs for the first time. Looking into my horse's eyes. Holding my wife's hand.

All of it. These moments froze in time as I marinated in the comfort they provided.

I have always said, "The little things are the big things in life," and I know this now more than ever.

Any issues or problems that happen in life now don't phase me. Why? Because nothing seems big in comparison to what I have experienced. For that, I am grateful.

I wouldn't change a thing.

I am so deeply grateful for the doctors, nurses, and treatments that saved my life.

I am so deeply grateful for my loved ones who stood by my side every step of the way.

I am so deeply grateful for ME.

Without my belief in myself, my commitment to LIVING, my courage, my will, and my passion for life, I wouldn't be here today.

Remember that no matter what, it comes down to you.

Recognize how powerful you are: your decisions, your spirit, your will, your heart, and your soul.

Take inventory of all the amazing things that make you, you: your strength, your love, your courage, and your resilience.

Gratitude begins with looking inward and appreciating all that you are.

You have everything you need inside of you, always.

To use this to overcome any challenge you must honor that, know that, and connect with that.

Gratitude is an anecdote to fear.

How many of you get paralyzed with fear in certain situations?

All of us have experienced fear.

Fear comes in many forms.

If we look at the fear experienced right before you are set to deliver an important presentation, conversation, or race, we can associate that fear with not wanting to fail.

Because if we fail, we will disappoint ourselves, the people we love, and everyone around us. If we disappoint these people, we fear losing their love or respect.

Yes, it goes that deep.

In an instant, you can change the meaning of something to positively influence your experience.

For instance, in that moment when you feel paralyzed with fear, you have a choice.

You can let that fear hold you back from giving everything you have toward being the best that you can be on that day.

Basically, you're protecting yourself.

If you don't fully put yourself out there, you won't put yourself in danger of failing. If you don't take big risks, you can feel safe and comfortable.

The problem is that the consequences of shrinking yourself to avoid failure are far worse than the consequences of taking a leap of faith, going all-in, and risking failure.

Why? Because if you don't lay it all out there, how will you ever know what you are truly capable of? How will you grow?

It is by going all IN, by taking risks, and tempting failure, that we grow.

When we fail, we learn. This is when we grow.

It is through problems or disappointment that we become connected to our greatest desires and what needs to be done to get from where we are to where we want to be.

If you sit back, don't risk at all, and let your fear hold you back from fully expressing your passion, the consequences are far more severe: feelings of inadequacy, stagnation, or weakness.

You'll create disappointment in yourself for not having the courage to step into the unknown. and see what you can do!

By letting your fear "bench you," you will never know just how far you can go, how fast you can go, or how tough you can be. You sit safely in the bud and will never fully bloom.

The moment we change the meaning of something, we create a lifelong transformation in our experiences.

Meaning leads to emotion. Emotion leads to action.

By changing the way we look upon how we feel just before "go time," we can change our entire experience of that event.

For instance, what if we took that feeling of fear and decided that it was just excitement? Excitement for the opportunity.

Excitement for the possibilities.

Generally, we feel fear because we care. We care about living up to our potential. We care about making all our hard work pay off. We care what other people think about us, and we care about people loving and respecting us.

But fear won't do us any good. It is a disempowering emotion.

Let's replace this fear with GRATITUDE.

When we feel gratitude, it is impossible to feel fear, anger, helplessness, or hatefulness at the same time.

Gratitude is by far the most empowering emotion that carries with it a meaning that can truly have you perform to the best of your ability.

Before any great challenge, or during it, I use gratitude to ground myself in a place where I can truly shine and where I feel empowered and positively inspired.

On race day, for example, this is what I would be present to:

1. I have been blessed with two arms, two legs, a strong heart, and the ability, opportunity, and desire to be out here partaking in a sport that I love.
2. I am doing something that makes me feel alive and that allows me to express my passion for pushing myself to my limits. It is an opportunity to grow and an opportunity to become more.
3. I am so lucky to be alive, to be experiencing a new place, and to be surrounded by other people that will stretch me. They will encourage me to find more within myself on this day.

These are three very simple thoughts that immediately put me in the most empowering state of gratitude.

The other thing that will help you step away from your fear, and step into your superhero costume, is realizing that if you give in to the fear, it will not lead you anywhere worth going.

If thinking a certain thought will only debilitate you, why would you CHOOSE to think that thought?

Fortune favors the bold.

The greater the risk, the greater the reward.

If you know that thinking positively leads to positive performance and feelings, but thinking negatively leads to negative performance and feelings, why would you choose anything but thinking positively?

Here is something to be grateful for: You have control over your thoughts. Your thoughts create your reality.

Be as disciplined with your thinking as you are with your work, training, or everyday responsibilities, and you will find that your experience of life is enhanced in the most beautiful ways.

Focus on what you want, not on what you don't want.

Focus on what you have, not what you don't have.

Focus on what is right, not on what is wrong.

This change of focus brings gratitude and appreciation.

In 2017, my greatest mentor asked me to speak at his Leadership Academy event.

I had never spoken in front of a crowd in my life except to receive my hall of fame induction in 2016.

But I can't say no to Tony Robbins. So, of course I said YES!

It was to be a ninety-minute slot. I was terrified.

I prepared hours on end for the two weeks before the event, writing pages and pages of thoughts, stories, and ideas to share.

When I would think about the actual event, I would freeze. This did not bode well for me.

Right before stage time, I was standing by the curtain hearing my name for my introduction. My palms were sweaty, my hands were shaking, and my heart was beating out of my chest.

I looked up to the sky, and I prayed. I prayed that I could be a gift to the two thousand beautiful souls attending the event. I prayed that I could be a blessing. I said a thank you for the humbling privilege of being asked to speak.

In gratitude and filled with a desire to serve everyone in the audience, I stepped on stage. I was ready.

I don't remember a thing I said in that ninety minutes. What I know is that it was not what I had rehearsed multiple times before that day. I spoke from my heart and focused only on what I could give to those people that would somehow make a difference in their lives.

Filled with gratitude, I was able to deliver a message that was received enthusiastically.

This is where my career of speaking on Tony Robbins's stages began. What a gift. What a blessing.

What a privilege.

From that point forward, every time before a speech, when I feel my sweaty palms and am winded by my pounding heart, shaking from the inside out, I know I am ready.

Ready to serve.

Ready to give my heart and soul.

Grateful for the opportunity.

As you step up to that thing that makes you fearful, acknowledge your fear, but then choose to step away from fear and into gratitude.

Turn up the volume on gratitude and mute the fear by dancing with it.

Bring it along with you and be grateful for the fact that this feeling means you care.

This feeling will keep you laser-focused on delivering to the best of your ability.

By creating an empowering meaning for all the feelings we have, we can change pain to pleasure, fear to inspiration, and disappointment to appreciation.

Commit to finding a higher level by finding a more empowering meaning for what you are feeling at all different times in life.

What can you appreciate?

This question always centers me in a way that leads me straight to gratitude.

Choose to forge forward with gratitude, and you will find your way through any challenge gracefully. You will fuel your actions with hope and energy that will guide you to achieve all that you hope.

Remember this:

- "Trade your expectation for appreciation, and see your entire world change in an instant"— Tony Robbins

- Change the way you look at things and the things you look at will change.

- Instead of thinking about how far you must go, think about how far you have come and feel grateful.

- So often our greatest victories come just around the corner of our biggest defeats.

- Gratitude is the bridge from despair to hope.

- Fortune favors the bold: with great risk comes great reward.

ASSIGNMENT: GRATITUDE HABITS

Gratitude is the most powerful energy source!

It is free energy and just takes going there to fill up.

Gratitude and thankfulness are linked to better health, greater happiness, stronger presence, better self-awareness, better relationships, more success, and greater fulfillment.

For the next seven days, I encourage you to participate in this ritual.

Morning Ritual:

First thing, when you open your eyes, write down or think about three things you are grateful for.

It could be as simple as "wow, I opened my eyes, and I can see. What a gift. I am so grateful."

It could be the cute doggie lying at the end of your bed or your partner lying next to you.

Really take in what is right, what is good, and what you can appreciate.

This starts your day with an abundance mindset, which will set you up for the best day possible.

Three things I am grateful for:

1.

2.

3.

Feel the gratitude.

If this is hard for you, try placing your hand on your beating heart. Feel the power, the strength, and the beauty of your heart. This is LIFE. The miraculous gift of life. Feel grateful.

Throughout the Day

Challenge yourself to ask the question: "What can I appreciate in this moment?"

This requires you to pause, reflect, and take in the feeling of gratitude.

List the three things that you must do every day that you don't enjoy.

1.

2.

3.

What can you appreciate about these things?

1.

2.

3.

Nighttime Ritual

Before you go to bed, go to the mirror and look yourself in the eyes.

Think about three things you love and appreciate about yourself.

Feel the appreciation for you.

Now, write down three things you are grateful for in your life or something that happened during the day that you are grateful for.

One at a time, think of each one and really feel the gratitude in your heart.

1.

2.

3.

Next, think about three WINS for the day.

What did you accomplish?
What did you overcome?
Did you make someone smile?
Did you make someone laugh?
Did you get a promotion?
Did you exercise longer than you
ever have and enjoyed it?
Did you get out of bed when you didn't feel like it?

A win is a win big or small. Celebrate it and be grateful for that good thing that happened or that thing you did that made you proud.

Chapter 7

THE POWER
OF INTENTION

*H*ow will you show up in your life today?

Doing things with intention gives you the power to create the experience you want to have.

In college, I used to wake up and say, "I hope today will be a good day," as if there was some greater force that determined whether I would be happy, sad, have a good game, or do well in my classes.

I went through my day hoping for the best and didn't put any intention into what I was going to do, thus creating the kind of day I hoped for.

You get to go first in deciding what experience you want to have every single day. You do this by deciding what to focus on, the meaning you give things, and the actions you decide to take.

I learned over time just how important meaning is in determining our future.

For example, if you lose your job, you can decide whether this means you no longer matter and will no longer be able to take care of yourself and others. Or you can decide that when one door closes, another door opens, and leads you to a much better place.

The things you MUST do in life I bet you don't enjoy doing them because you HAVE to do them. What if you changed the language to "I get to" do these things?

The meaning we give things sets us up for what it will be like to experience doing them.

Working out is something I LOVE. It makes me feel alive. It centers me. It is like therapy for me. I feel free. I feel invigorated. I feel strong and confident once I finish.

The meaning I give it serves me well. It sees me waking up excited to exercise every single morning.

What if you hate working out? Working out is hard. Working out is exhausting. Working out hurts. I HAVE to work out if I want to be healthy. If you give it this unflattering meaning, surely, it will be hard to get yourself to do it.

Create awareness around the things you HAVE to do. What meaning do you give these things? Change the meaning to something you GET to do. Change the meaning to something that inspires you to do it. Suddenly, you are not only consistently doing that thing but taking great pleasure in doing so.

We can look at the dishes in the sink as a chore that we hate, or we can look at dishes as something we are so blessed to have. Having a sink full of dishes means we have enough food on the table to share with many people.

Say you have lots of laundry to wash. How lucky are you that you don't have to wear the same outfit every day because that's all you have? A big load of laundry means you have the good fortune of being able to choose a different outfit each day. It means you can clothe your children and your family. What a blessing.

Can you see how just shifting the meaning you give things can completely change your feelings about it?

It's time to be your own biggest supporter and choose to find joy in the mundane chores you are faced with each day.

Find joy in daily routines like working out, eating healthy, or cleaning the house by reframing what those things mean to you.

Here is how you go about setting yourself up to have the best experience with everything you do.

Ask yourself: What do I want to experience?

For example: I want to enjoy this workout and get the most out of it.

Okay, so next question: to experience that, how must I show up?

I know that exercise will improve my mood and give me energy to take into the rest of my day. I will stay present to the benefits of moving my body and feel grateful for the strength, health, and ability I have to do so.

You're going into an important meeting where you will be presenting to your team.

What do you want to experience?

I want to feel confident and ready, focused solely on delivering my content from my heart with energy, passion, clarity, and authenticity.

Okay, so how do you need to show up?

I need to show up fully present, not thinking about that one time I messed up and not thinking about how awful it would be if I mess up again in the future.

I will be fully present in the moment, tapping into my highest potential to deliver what I have inside of me. I will show up prepared, energized, and grateful for the opportunity.

Can you see how doing things intentionally can set you up for a much better experience?

This puts it all in your capable hands. You get to create an experience where you can optimize what you are able to deliver and the impact that will have.

Intention is about taking who you know you are and bringing it into the world.

Whatever you want more of in life, you must go first in being that.

You want more romance? Be more romantic.

You want more appreciation? Be more appreciative.

You want more love? Be more loving. It is only by giving love that we are loved.

You want more joy? Be more joyful.

You want more energy? Do more things that energize you!

Be intentional about bringing what you want into the world. It starts with you.

When I got leukemia, everyone was telling me what I was going to experience. You will be so sick. You will have no energy. You won't get out of bed for at least a month after your bone marrow transplant. I was not going to take someone else's experience and live the same one.

I didn't want that to be my truth. So, I decided to create my own experience.

If I had the energy to run while on treatment, I would run.

If I could walk on the treadmill the day after my bone marrow transplant, then I would walk. And I did!

I was intentional about the fact that I would keep moving as much as I could during my treatment and recovery. Why? Because walking and moving my body gave me energy, made me feel strong and alive, and it was what I wanted. This is what I needed so I could have the confidence to find my way through the sickness, pain, and suffering and out the other side to triumph.

I didn't want to take on the fear of chemo and radiation. People talked of the "poison taking over their body." If I chose to look at it that way, I feel I would have suffered even more than I was. Instead, right before the chemo was injected into my blood, I would say a small prayer, "Thank you for healing me. Thank you for coming into my body to kill the cancer and deliver me to health. I am so deeply grateful."

Just by giving the chemo this meaning, it made me fear it less. In accepting it as the healing agent it was, I set myself up for a much more bearable experience with less stress and less emotional suffering.

I was intentional about wanting to leave no stone unturned to ensure my survival.

At the start of my treatment, my dear friend Mary Gerdts came out to spend a couple days with me. I am so deeply grateful for all her guidance in preparing me for the road ahead. It was so deeply powerful. Oftentimes, it was extremely uncomfortable but so empowering.

We spoke about how things like resentment, anger, regret, sadness, and angst all cause dis-ease. Through our work together, I committed to releasing any anger, pain, or resentment that resided within me. In doing this, I would effectively sweep out my soul, making room for the healing to move through me.

Any moment I had a thought about something I regretted, or someone that had hurt me or let me down, I would sit with it to feel the emotion and find compassion for myself, or for the other person. Forgive and let go.

This was a very intentional process. With each resolution, I felt lighter. I felt cleansed, and I felt ready to receive the treatment that I prayed would save my life.

How do you look at your failures?

If you let them knock you down, steal your thunder, demoralize you and strip you of your confidence, you will avoid failure at all costs. This will lead you to play it safe and not do a lot of the things you dream of doing.

Be intentional about how you will handle failure should it find you.

I chose to see failure as an incredible opportunity to learn, which would then equip me with further knowledge or insight that would encourage more progress toward my goal.

The meaning I gave failure was learning.

I was either winning, which I defined as making progress, or I was learning.

Every day, I intentionally directed my thoughts around my experiences in this way, which led to me never losing hope, giving up, or giving in. It led to me always find a way to progress.

You can use intention to manage the difficult relationships in your life.

Who can relate to the stress and dread leading into major holidays where you know you will be getting together with family?

For many years, Christmas was something I looked forward to, coming home and spending time with my mom and seeing my sister. The visions in my mind would include lots of hugs and laughs, and great conversations over one of my mom's legendary, delicious culinary creations.

The hugs came. The laughs. The incredible food. But then always, the subject would come up about my sister's drinking, and this beautiful dream-like holiday turned into a war zone.

Yelling and screaming and my mom's tears. My anger would well up inside of me like a tire being pumped up with air so much that you could hear it leaking through the sides, warning you that if any more came in, it would POP.

I couldn't stand the fact that my sister, once again, was ruining Christmas.

Here's the thing: my sister didn't ruin Christmas all those years. I did.

I told myself when these fights would start that this was RUINING Christmas. But was it really?

My response, my reaction to whatever triggered the fight, was in my control. But I didn't control it. Without saying a word, my energy spoke volumes and would heighten the emotions barreling into the room.

I could have responded differently. I could have been intentional about creating a wonderful Christmas or intentional about DECIDING that one argument will not ruin Christmas.

One argument would be just one argument, and we would move through it the best that we could and then come back to take in the beautiful meal that my mom would inevitably create.

When we EXPECT to experience certain things at certain times, we almost go in looking for it, waiting for it to happen. It is in the anticipation of this occurring that our energy shifts and we invite it in, proving ourselves right. What we expected to happen, did.

Using intention, I decided I no longer wanted to dread Christmas.

I wanted to celebrate the divine holiday and make great memories—memories that would ultimately shift the paradigm of emotions leading into it in the future.

I decided to use something that I use at work: choose to see whomever it is you are working with as the best version of themselves and go into a meeting expecting the very best from them, not the worst.

This leads to you giving off an energy of acceptance, respect, and love. This energy will be felt by the other person and they in kind will show up, more likely as the higher version of themselves.

Don't go in with expectations about what will or will not happen.

Go in intending to appreciate. Appreciate all that is right. All that is good.

Appreciate the best qualities of the people you will be around.

If you don't have expectations, you won't be disappointed.

If you don't have expectations, you are more likely to find things to appreciate.

The first Christmas I decided to be intentional ended up being the most wonderful Christmas of my life.

It came just days after my diagnosis. I was unwilling to experience any more pain than what I was already feeling. The pain of uncertainty. The pain of fear and worry and anticipation of the long and scary road ahead.

My wife and I showed up at my mom's adorable house where we would have dinner with my sister, mom, and all our dogs! (Seven between the four of us.)

I said to Bek before going in, "I love my sister. I am going to focus on all the things I love about her. Her big loving heart, her sense of humor, her kindness. I will see her and treat her as that person that I see."

In the past, I would focus solely on how drunk she was, how she was treating my mom, and all she had taken or would take in the future. I would tense up before even walking through the door.

We walked in and had the most beautiful night. I looked into my sister's eyes and saw her deep pain. She was locked in a cycle that she couldn't get out of. I felt compassion. I felt a profound love for my sister who sat with tears in her eyes, telling me how much she loved me and wanted me to live.

I could feel her heart expanding out to hold mine. I could feel her care. I could feel her love. I could feel her presence, and I saw her for who she really is, not the label I had tacked onto her.

My mom made the most amazing meal and set the table in the way she always does—beautiful, charming touches that made me want to just freeze time in that moment of being present to the beautiful gift of the day.

We spoke of how I would triumph, how we would all come together to make a miracle.

I saw my sister, and she felt seen. She felt understood. She felt supported and so did I.

This created the most wonderful memory—a memory that laid the groundwork for every other holiday that came after it.

How can you show up differently to events that often bring out the worst in you?

Maybe you find it hard being around people that are negative.

The people that scoff at your dreams or try to dim your light.

Here is my advice and this requires INTENTION:

BE THE EAGLE

The only other bird that tries to mess with the eagle is the black crow.

As the eagle flies, the black crow comes and nips at the eagle's wings, trying to get it to fall to the ground.

What the eagle does is he flies higher and higher and higher until he reaches an altitude where the black crow can no longer fly. So, the crow falls back, and the eagle continues to soar.

Take the high road. Be the eagle for you and as an example for others.

Remember this:

- Change "I have to" to "I get to" and see your entire experience change.

- Before any meeting or practice, be intentional:

    o What do I want to experience?
    o How do I need to show up?

- You can do anything with intention.

- Whatever you want more of in your life, go first in giving that.

- Be the EAGLE!

ASSIGNMENT: INTENTIONALITY

WEEKLY INTENTION PLANNER

SELF

Three words that describe my best self are:

1.

2.

3.

Here are some ideas for how I can embody these words more often this coming week:

SOCIAL

Three words defining how I want to treat other people this week:

1.

2.

3.

Some people in my life with whom I can improve my interactions are:

SKILLS

The five skills I am working on developing most in my life right now are:

1.

2.

3.

4.

5.

What are the ways I can practice those skills this week?

SERVICE AND CONTRIBUTION

What are three small things I can do to add value to someone else this week?

1.

2.

3.

What can I do today or this week with presence, focus, and excellence to help someone?

FEELINGS

The main feelings I want to cultivate in my life, relationships, self, and work this week are:

What can I do to generate those feelings more every day?

Define what is most meaningful in life:

What can I do or create that would give my life more meaning?

Chapter 8

THE POWER
OF PRESENCE

*T*he next stop along the Power Line is Presence.
We are most powerful when we are fully present—not
sitting in the pain of the past and not obsessing over
worries of the future, just being fully there in the moment and
opening our eyes to the magic that is within us and around us.

Presence leads to more powerful work being done, deeper
and more fulfilling relationships, and a greater understanding
of how very blessed we are in our lives.

So many people talk about feeling overwhelmed by working full-time, being a mom or a dad, and the many responsibilities involved. When they ask me how to deal with this
overwhelming feeling, my first piece of advice is to practice presence.

When you are at work, focus solely on what you are doing
in every moment.

Laser focus on the moment. This will see you accomplish
your work more efficiently and effectively. By being present,
you can truly bring your best work to fruition.

Then, when it is time to get home and be with family, put your phone away, put your work aside, and be fully present with your family. Truly listen to how their day was. Be there with them, fully present.

Even if you only have an hour of time to spend together, if you are fully present, that hour will bring even more fulfillment and closeness than five hours together while you're distracted by work, your phone, and worrying about the future.

I will never forget the 2010 Ironman World Championship.

I was coaching my athlete, Mirinda Carfrae, whose goal was to WIN the world championship the following day.

I was so nervous and trying to put together my pre-race talk that I would deliver to her the evening before the race.

Trying to figure out a way to calm my nerves, I decided to go into a hot yoga class that I passed on my walk home.

I had never done yoga before, but I was drawn to join on that day.

Everyone around me seemed to be very well-versed in this practice, standing like statues while I wobbled all over the place.

In trying to find the balance necessary to hold a pose, I decided to just clear my mind and focus only on what I was doing in that very moment.

Once I got present and focused only on what was necessary to achieve that balance, I stood and became a statue myself, solid and grounded as if I had done this for years.

What I was searching for was delivered in a beautifully wrapped-up package with a ribbon on the top. My advice to Mirinda before the race would be this:

Be fully present in the moment. In every single moment. Just focus on every single swim stroke, pedal stroke, and running step. You are most powerful when you are fully present in the moment. String together as many moments as you can in this state and every ounce of your ability will lead the way.

The next day, she did just that, focusing on her and her alone and doing the best that she could in every moment. Not focusing on what happened in the last moment. Not focusing on what could go wrong in the next moment. Just in the moment. Every single moment. She won her first Ironman World Championship that day.

Tell me this, what would you prefer: five hours with your loved one together in the same room but both of you playing on your phones, taking work calls, or watching TV? Or thirty minutes just being together, talking, listening, fully present with one another?

Which scenario do you think would make you feel more seen, heard, and understood?

Which scenario do you think would fill you up and bring you closer together?

Presence.

Think about the hockey player, skating down the ice with the puck. If he/she is thinking about the last time they missed the cage, or what will happen if they miss the cage in the future, they will not score the goal. What will give this player the best chance at scoring is being present in that moment.

The grip on the stick, the look to the cage, the power put into the swing, and BOOM, score!

Presence.

You are headed into work to give a presentation.

If you focus on the last time you presented and it didn't go well, or what it would feel like in the future if you fail, do you think you will give a great presentation?

Probably not.

Be present. Deliver from your heart. Stand tall. Believe in yourself and just do your thing.

I assure you the results will be what you hope for!

To know what we want most in life, we must be present with who we are. What things make you feel most alive? What inspires you? What drains you, or makes you feel bad?

What are your deepest desires?

Being able to answer these things requires you to be present with yourself.

This is the KEY.

Don't just push your emotions or feelings away as they will build up, fester, and come back to haunt you.

It is so important to feel your feelings. Label them. Get curious as to why you feel that way. And get curious about what you can do to feel better, move beyond whatever is causing you pain, and find a better way.

You cannot know where you want to go in life if you don't stop and think about where you are, what you want, and how you will best get there.

This requires presence.

Be present with you. Step into your authentic power. Embrace all of who you are. Back yourself!

Advocate for yourself.

Be there for yourself.

Don't ignore your feelings.

Don't abandon yourself.

Step up for yourself.

Loving yourself and OWNING yourself is a powerful predictor of successful relationships and a fulfilling life.

We cannot skip that step, and it starts with presence.

Presence can be that ONE thing that breaks unhealthy patterns in relationships.

My sister, Lisa, has had a lifelong battle with alcoholism and bulimia.

Since the age of sixteen, she has put her body through wars. At fifty-five years old, her body finally started shutting down, dropping to eighty-four pounds and losing her spirit to live.

I had witnessed her decline for a long while but just this past year, it became obvious that her habits were killing her, and THIS was killing my mom.

My mom was taking all the blame. She felt like she had somehow failed my sister.

My mom put the responsibility on herself to somehow make everything okay.

For so many years I felt anger: anger that Lisa couldn't just turn herself around, become responsible, take ownership of her mistakes, and vow to do better.

Maybe I lived in this space to somehow protect myself. My own feelings. My own life. But what I realize now was that this was unfair. Not just to her, but to me.

Who was I to judge her actions when I hadn't taken the time to be present enough with her to understand her pain?

Empathy is being able to put yourself in someone else's shoes and imagine what they might be feeling or thinking.

Empathy requires presence.

Empathy requires listening.

When I got AML, I was in dire need of a matching donor. Thankfully, my sister was a perfect match. My mom was a match as well. I felt so deeply blessed to know this. The doctors wanted me to go with Lisa's cells due to her being closer to my age.

My biggest fear was that on the day of the transplant, she wouldn't show up. She would be off somewhere drunk, forget about the fact that she said she would save me, and not show up.

My sister would NEVER do that.

My sister loved me and finally, she was being given a responsibility that meant so much to her.

She was being given an opportunity to save my life. To be my hero.

Giving me life gave my sister great purpose. The gift she gave me, I realize, was a gift for her as well.

As I continued to take steps toward healing, fighting to win the battle against AML, my sister continued her battle with the lifelong demons of alcohol and bulimia.

Where I had a team of experts around me, doing everything they could to save my life, my sister had her family around her but all of us with no clue how to help.

For so long, I had felt such sadness and frustration over the burden my sister's behaviors had on my mom.

Couldn't my sister just get her stuff together to remove some of the pressure and anxiety?

With her bone marrow donation, along with that of a generous umbilical cord, came a new thought and a new perspective. If I can be given life as a fifty-year-old, when it seems impossible, can't anyone be given a new chance at life? At any time? What would have to happen?

For so long, I had focused on how she was hurting us with her reckless behaviors.

I was so focused on how she was hurting us that I never took the time to see how much she loved us. She wasn't doing these things to hurt us. She was doing these things because it was all she knew. This was how she had learned to cope. Having done this for so long, she was caught in this raging current with no life preserver in sight.

My mom had tried all kinds of different programs to help her. She never gave up but at the same time, she was exhausted trying. Lisa seemed unwilling to assist in her own recovery and unwilling to do the work necessary to overcome decades of bad habits.

For her, life had been so hard. Battling these demons was so, so hard. She was exhausted and had no "try" left to beat the gigantic monster that was raging out of control.

Yes, we were trying to take her places to "fix" her.

Until she got what she really needed most, she would not be fixable.

What did she really need?

I believe it was presence, understanding, listening, and empathy.

These things led to her talking more about what she had to contend with in her mind every second of every day. Talking about it lessened the shame. This shame was the sting in every action she took, driving her to fall deeper into the chasm of pain.

Why had I not done this earlier? Where had I been?

Locked in judgment. Watching and waiting for her to somehow find a way.

The door blocking the way was missing the key.

I vowed to spend more time with my sister, to be intentional about seeing my sister as her highest self: the loving, kind, compassionate, but deeply suffering woman that she was.

As I showed up looking for the best in her, all I found was her loving, caring, beautiful heart.

I would listen to her as she spoke from her heart. How lost she felt. How crazy she felt. How out of control. I listened, truly listened, without judgment. I opened my heart, so moved by her, so deeply affected by her pain.

Human beings are all hardwired for empathy but often we fail in giving it because of our own pain. For so long, I was in pain watching my sister not only destroy her own life but take the people I loved most down with her.

I needed to step out of my own way and be there for her. I needed to better understand her. See her. Be with her in the space of her truth lovingly, with acceptance, compassion, and empathy.

When we are willing to fully listen, the depth of understanding and meaning we receive brings a greater depth and trust to the relationship.

By meeting another with compassion and understanding, you are giving them the most nourishing gift.

Presence can lead you to see someone different than you previously had. This will give you the opportunity to respond differently, forging a new path that can lead to resolution.

In February of 2022, as my sister's body was failing her and her mind going along with it, she had written a suicide note. Thankfully, her roommate found it before anything happened. When we found my sister, we admitted her immediately to the ICU, where she stayed for two weeks.

From there she moved to three different drug and alcohol treatment centers. She successfully stopped drinking, but the bulimia continued. No one felt they had the capacity to care for someone as sick as she was. They were afraid for their own reputations and liability.

Desperate to save her daughter's life, my mom spent every hour of every day trying to find a place that would admit my sister and at least TRY to save her.

By this point, Lisa was merely an empty shell. She was eighty-five pounds and in and out of hospitals due to life-threateningly low sodium and potassium levels.

Now that she was sober, all her mental and emotional anguish went into the bulimia. She just couldn't stop on her own. She needed help from a place that specialized in this. No one would take her.

My mom would call five to six places a day. After spending $30,000 per month for four months already, she was trying to find a place that would take Medicaid. My mom was ready to sell her house—to do whatever had to be done to save her daughter's life.

I was so deeply touched by the strength, will, and determination my mom showed which was all driven by her love for my sister. But I also knew that the only person that could save my sister was my sister.

What needed to happen for her to WANT to get better? For her to finally back herself?

Presence was required in every moment.

Empathy.

We must try to understand so that somehow we can help, even with just the gift of listening.

At one point, I had to ask her, "Lisa, do you want to live? I know how deeply you are suffering. I feel your pain.

Your body somehow has withstood the most horrific war for thirty-nine years. This extraordinary body of yours has never ever given up. Have you thought about how incredible this body of yours is? Still standing after all you have put it through.

Don't you want to step up for this loyal and devoted body and do your part?

It is time now for you to be the hero of your body.

For thirty-nine years your body has been fighting to live despite you hammering it with alcohol and bulimia. It's like your body is riding the tandem bike, doing all the pedaling as you sit back and trash it. You must start carrying some of the load. You must start pedaling.

Only you can be the hero of your own life.

You have been my hero, you have been your dog's hero, but now it is time for you."

I could tell she listened, but I was unsure if it resonated deep enough.

So, the next day, with my throat locked up in anticipation, I said what needed to be said. "Lisa, if you keep throwing up when your body is hanging on by a thread, then we need to discuss your will. Where do you want to be buried, what would you like me to say? Because if you don't change anything, you will die. It could be a matter of days." I held back tears as I said these words that shocked me as I spoke them.

I needed to try to make this real for her.

Her body was shutting down, and it was killing us to see it happening.

"I love you with all my heart, Lisa. I want to have a future together with you."

Now that we had connected so deeply through presence and empathy, I so desperately wanted a second chance to live life with a sister. To love her. To elevate her. To share life together.

"I don't want to die," she said.

I cried.

I said, "Lisa, if you get into a place that can help you, you must do the work.

You must do whatever they ask you to do.

You must participate in your own rescue, and this requires you to believe that you can do the hard work and make it through to the other side."

When I was told how I was going to fight AML, I couldn't pick and choose what parts I would do and what parts I wouldn't. I was going to do WHATEVER it took to survive. I was ALL IN! It was a matter of living or dying.

Lisa needed to be willing to do the same.

Talking about her funeral, I believe, is what shifted her perspective. After months of resisting treatment, she now said she was ready. She wanted help.

The next day, after six months of rejection after rejection, my mom received a phone call from a place in Utah accepting Lisa for treatment.

Before my mom and Lisa drove off, I asked Lisa how she felt and she answered, "I am excited."

The smile on my lips and the smile in my heart left me speechless. For the first time in thirty-nine years, I FELT the truth in her words.

She was ready, and I believed in her.

My sister was now willing to become the hero of her own life.

Don't wait for someone to be who you want them to be, or where you want them to be.

Meet them where they are.

Love them where they are.

What can you learn about them? What can you learn from them?

Listen. Lean in. Be present and give empathy.

Now that I know better, I do better. I only wish it didn't take me this long.

Do you have a loved one that is struggling? Do you have someone in your life that you no longer are connected to because they are living life in a way you don't agree with?

If you want to resolve this relationship, or at least resolve the pain it causes you within, I encourage you to meet them with a different perspective.

Leave your beliefs and judgment at the door.

Sit down with the intention to listen.

To try to better understand how they feel and what they are thinking.

Just being seen, heard, and better understood can lead to deep healing.

It sure did with my sister and me. It brought us closer together than ever before.

I saw HER. Not her as she related to who I thought she should be, or how I thought she should live her life. Just her. Lisa Lindley. My sister. A human being who was lost, suffering, and needed help. Help in the form of presence. Help in the form of empathy.

Bring empathy. Be present.

Bring you, all of you, and let the healing begin.

Presence is the way to a deeper connection.

Presence is the way to optimize your full potential.

Presence is the way to knowing yourself, what you are feeling, what you are needing, and what you must do to experience what you hope to in any given moment.

This must be conditioned. Practiced daily. It's worth the practice, so let's get started now.

Remember:

- Do not judge people, instead, try to understand them.

- Remember to feel your feelings.

- Empathy: put yourself in someone else's shoes.

- Presence leads to more powerful work being done, deeper and more fulfilling relationships, and lower anxiety and stress.

- Presence with self is a requirement for living authentically and finding your way.

- Presence may be that one vital ingredient that leads to the resolution you are searching for.

ASSIGNMENT: THE POWER OF PRESENCE

Here is your goal: GO ALL IN in every moment, present and grounded, and see your entire experience of life deepen in the most beautiful and powerful ways.

So, how can you do this? Start with this:

Make the DECISION to be intentional about being present.

"I am going to be more intentional in every interaction with my partner."

We will start with just one aspect of your life—it can be deciding to be more present with your husband or wife. Or deciding to be more present while working on a distinct project.

Once you decide what area of life you will focus on, relationships, self, career, or health, commit to seven days of being intentional about it.

What area of your life will you decide to be more present in?

Pick three parts of your day when you spend time with your spouse, loved ones, or yourself that you know that you are not fully present and write those down using the worksheet attached. Under each part, write down the things that you are doing or thinking about instead of being present.

Then follow the same process with other areas of your life where you could be more present, such as work or time with yourself.

1. *Enter the first situation with your loved one here.*

What normally distracts you?

2. *Enter the second situation with your loved one here.*
   What normally distracts you?

3. *Enter the third situation with your loved one here.*
   What normally distracts you?

AWARENESS IS KEY:

Tomorrow, during those times of the day, you are going to make a conscious effort to be fully present and not be distracted by any of those things you noted.

What must you do differently?

What will you no longer do during those times together?

Example:

My wife and I love to spend time together at dinner. We share stories about our day and connect deeply. Sometimes, however, I have lingering work responsibilities on my mind. Because of that, I keep my phone nearby and even if I don't pick it up, I am looking over at it, constantly thinking about how many emails and messages are piling up.

This leads me to not being present for my wife, and her feeling ignored.

So, with this exercise, I would plan to leave my phone in the other room out of sight and energetically commit to detaching from work and being fully present for my wife.

It takes two people to successfully create this presence. So, have a conversation with your loved one and decide together to leave your phones in another room.

At the end of the day, write down how it went, what went well, and what didn't go so well.

What could you do differently?

How can you improve upon the experience the next time?

1. *Enter the first situation you are working at being more present for.*
   What went well?
   What didn't go well?
   What should you do differently next time?

2. *Enter the second situation you are working at being more present for.*
   What went well?
   What didn't go well?
   What should you do differently next time?

3. *Enter the third situation you are working at being more present for.*
   What went well?
   What didn't go well?
   What should you do differently next time?

What did you find was the best part of being present?

What did you notice about the interactions you had?

If you were present with your work, did you feel more effective? Did you work more efficiently?

Stack the evidence for the power of presence so that you can see the importance of it and aim to be present in as many moments as possible.

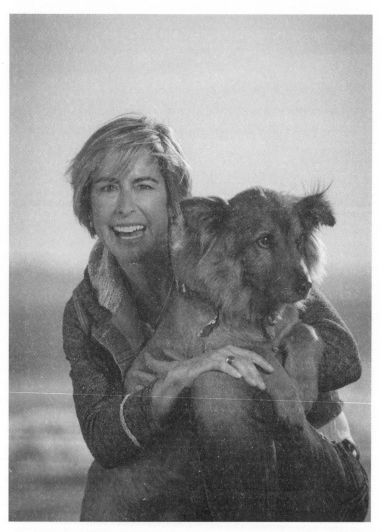

Calvin, my soulmate doggie that I learned so much from.

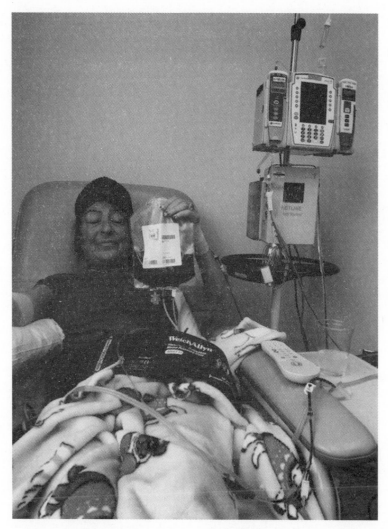

My sister who, together with a donor umbilical cord, gave me life!

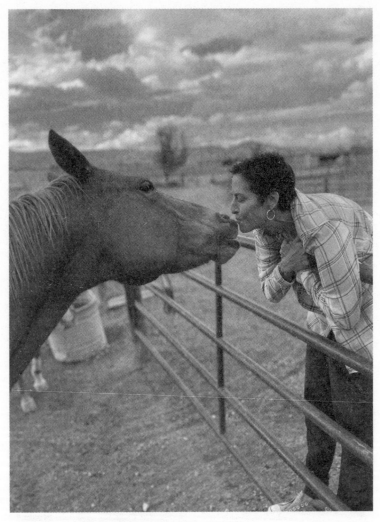

Savannah: Developing a relationship with her
changed me at the deepest levels.

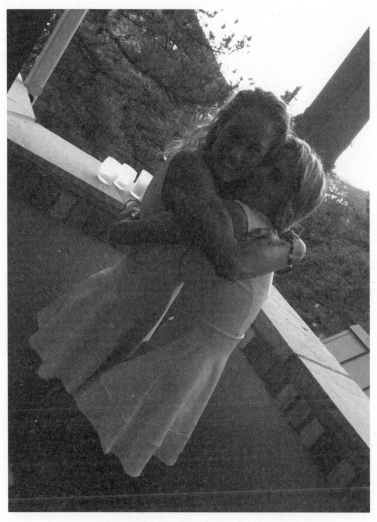

Bek, the love of my life. Finally, I found love and loved
myself enough to trust in her love for me.

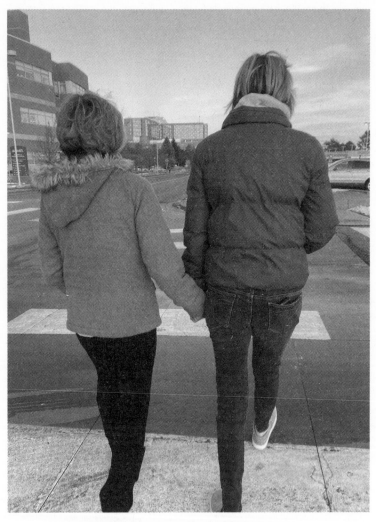

Mom: Always by my side through my toughest times.
My rock. My best friend. My biggest cheerleader.

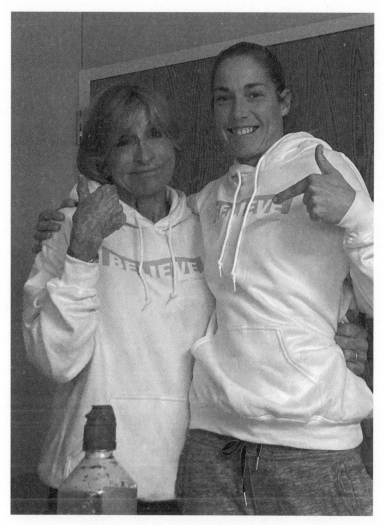

Mom brought my dogs to visit me during my long stay
in hospital, pre-bone marrow transplant. She slept on
the couch every single night for thirty nights.

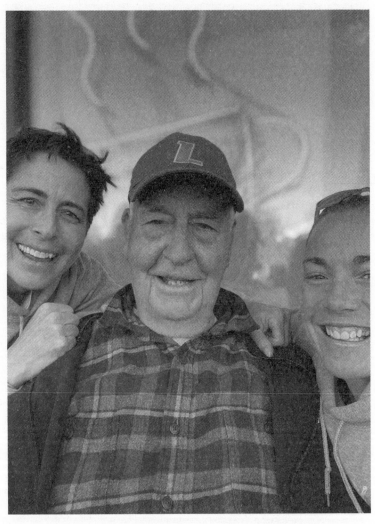

Dad: We have been through so much. Forgiveness has
brought us back together—stronger than ever.

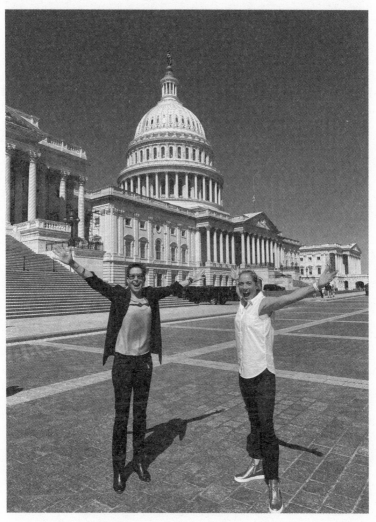

Advocating for horses around the world.

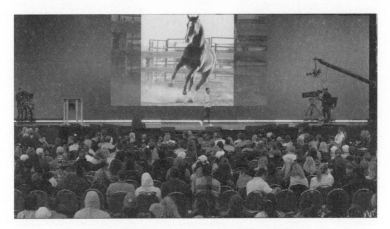

Me on stage sharing my story of rescuing
Savannah from the slaughter pipeline.

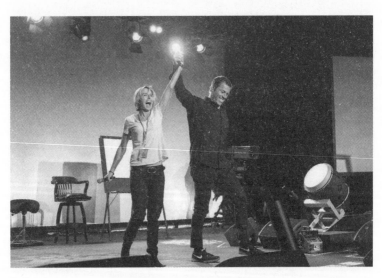

On stage with my greatest mentor, Tony Robbins, twenty-seven
years after first becoming a student of his teachings. So guided.

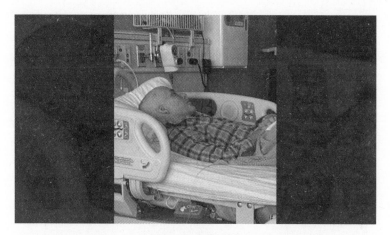

Fighting for my life.

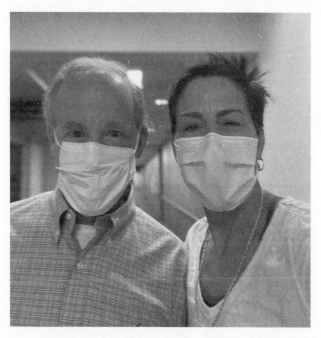

Dr. Gutman who, along with Dr. Pollyea, saved my life through
their clinical trials and extraordinary care. Forever grateful to
them and all my nurses and staff at UC Health Anschutz.

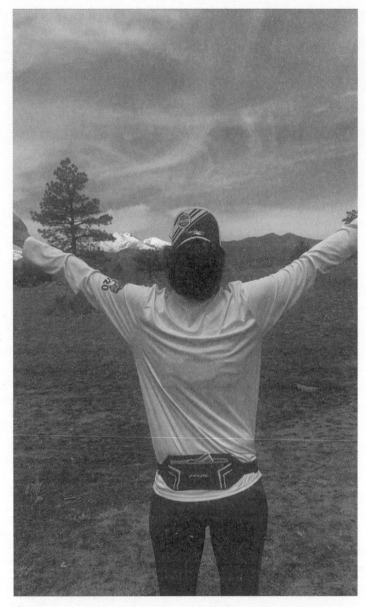

One year post-bone marrow transplant running my favorite mountain. "I am cancer free! I get to live! Praise God!"

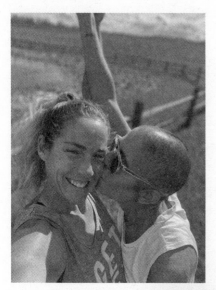

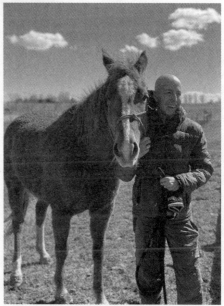

Able to return home after two months away for bone marrow transplant. The joy I felt was immeasurable.

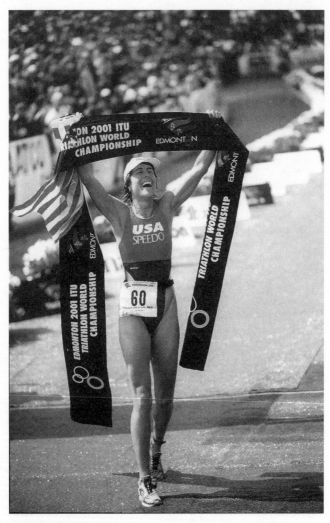

Winning the World Championship 2001: The day I proved
that what seems impossible is really possible.

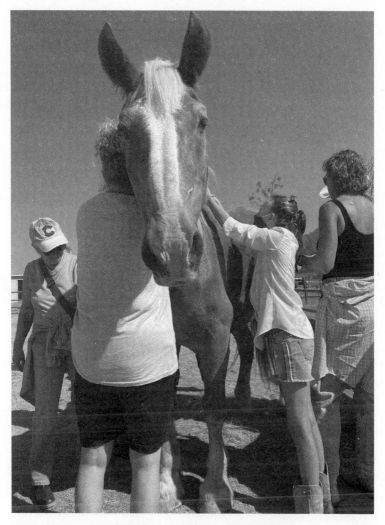

Equine Assisted Healing events at Believe
Ranch and Rescue facilitated by me.

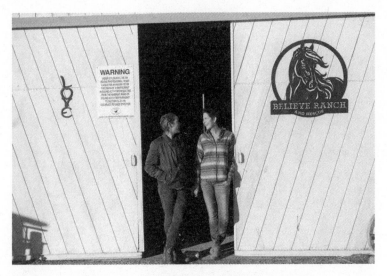

Believe Ranch and Rescue: To date, we have
saved 252 horses from slaughter.

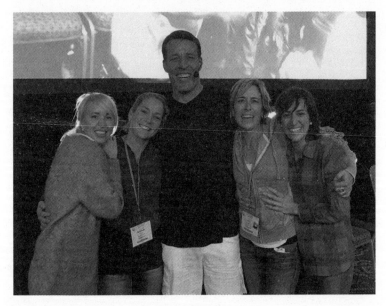

Chosen family.

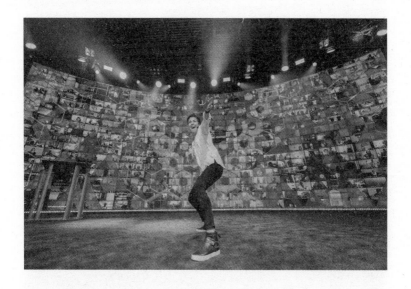

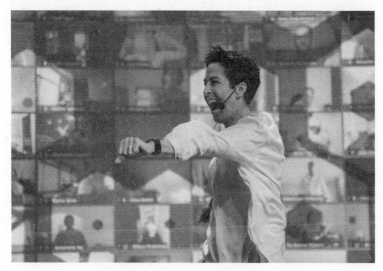

Living my mission and purpose. So blessed to
speak on my greatest mentor's stage!

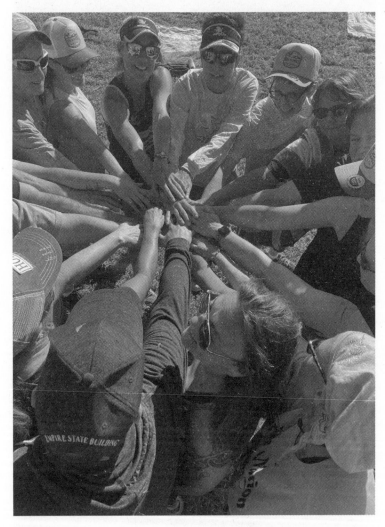

Sirius Squad

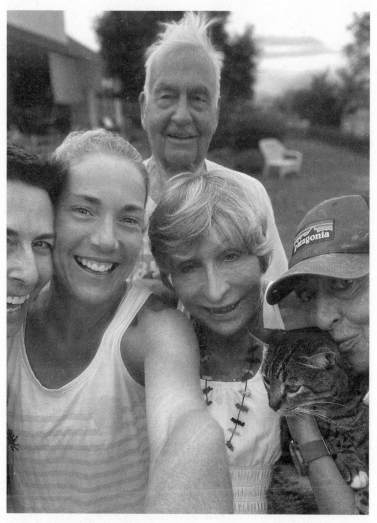

Bringing the family together to celebrate my triumph.

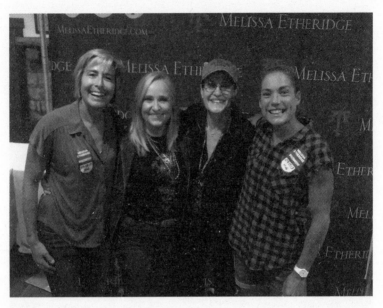

The day forever friends were made, July 2019.

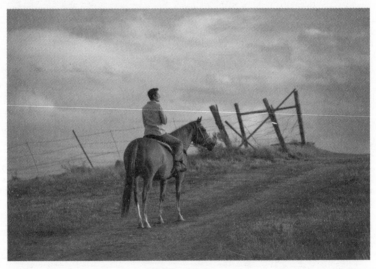

Forever grateful.

Chapter 9

THE POWER
OF PURPOSE

*W*hat does living with purpose mean to you?

My purpose in life is to live fully, love with all my heart, and make a beautiful difference in as many humans' and animals' lives as I can.

I want to guide people like you HOME, to the magic within you.

I stand up for humans and animals. Help them find their voice.

My deep desire is to help you live your best life: the life you were destined to live. I want to guide you home to your authentic self and empower you to take the reins so you can create the life you dream of in every moment.

My purpose and mission fueled me during the darkest times of my illness.

In 2019, Bek and I organized an incredible gala to raise money for our nonprofit 501(c)(3), Horses in Our Hands. Our goal was to raise $500,000 to fund our national campaign, raising awareness of the horrific brutal slaughter of horses. In raising awareness, we could amplify our voices and be heard by Washington, DC. In doing this, our goal was to pass the SAFE Act (Save America's Forgotten Equines), which would end this horrific practice once and for all.

The gala was scheduled for March 1, eight days after my bone marrow transplant on February 20.

Bek wanted to cancel the whole thing, saying she couldn't leave me during such a crucial time.

There was NO WAY we were going to cancel what would be the most impactful event for our work as a nonprofit.

We had been working tirelessly to not only save those beautiful horses from slaughter but also on developing the content, strategy, vision, and outcomes for what would happen next.

I promised they could call me in on Zoom, and I would present to the best of my ability on the night.

We had the most incredible turnout at Calamigos Ranch in Malibu, California.

Our greatest supporters attended, like Tony Robbins and his wife Sage; Mary Gerdts; Julianne Hough, who performed that evening; Smokey Robinson; John Paul DeJoria; and Melissa Etheridge, who played all night long.

It was an incredible evening. We were educating beautiful people about the horrors of what was happening to those majestic beings.

I called in from my hospital bed, so weak, and very sick. Nothing would stop me from presenting on that night. This mission meant everything to me, and I would follow through no matter what.

We raised $500,000 that night, and since then, have used that money to educate over eighty-four million homes about the brutality of horse slaughter through a national commercial we had made.

Our social media campaign was unlike anything other major animal groups had done in the past.

We had 250 thousand emails sent to legislators asking them to pass the SAFE Act and

1,800 letters to the editors of major news outlets.

We have decreased the number of horses being sent to slaughter from sixty thousand in 2019 to twenty-six thousand in 2022—a major reduction thanks to our awareness campaign.

Keep in mind, when my wife and I said that we were going to ban slaughter altogether, people laughed at us. They said we only had horses for five years. How could you accomplish something that no one else, even the Humane Society and the American Society for the Prevention of Cruelty to Animals (ASPCA), haven't been able to do for twenty years?

Change your story. Change your life.

We were NOT willing to live the story that said because we had no experience with horses, there was no chance we could ban slaughter.

NO. We told ourselves that because we were world-class athletes, whose superpowers are endurance, grit, and relentlessness, we would not stop until we passed the SAFE Act. Or, until we found some way to end this brutal practice once and for all.

After three years of nonstop raising-awareness campaigns, lobbying in DC, and connecting with most members of the House of Representatives and Senate, Bek and I moved this bill further than it had gotten in twenty years. At the time of writing this, October 2022, the bill is being discussed in Colloguy with key legislators to find a way to pass this congress.

One of the strongest groups of opposition has been the AVMA the American Veterinary Medical Association. They claim that horse slaughter is humane euthanasia. This is absolutely untrue. So, we gathered footage from slaughterhouses in Canada and Mexico, taken by Animals' Angels, a nonprofit that exposes animal abuse.

We put together footage and flew to Washington, D.C. to set the record straight with Congress people and Senate members. We sat down in dozens of offices and showed a video of the reality of this horrific practice.

At the time of writing this, the bill is awaiting markup from the Energy and Commerce Committee.

Key Horse advocates like Chairman Frank Pallone and Senator Bob Menendez are doing whatever they can to find a way to either pass the SAFE Act or find another way to ban this practice altogether.

Politics is not for the faint of heart. This journey has been so very emotional for me. Stripping me down to the rawest emotions of frustration, overwhelm, despair, and sadness. Highs and lows. One day we'll get filled with hope as more and more members sign their support of banning horse slaughter and then the next day, another big group comes out in opposition.

Those opposed have been misinformed in regard to what they know about horse slaughter.

We have debunked every myth and set the record straight on our website www.horsesinourhands.org.

As we raise awareness around the globe, we have thankfully inspired celebrities like Bella Hadid, who has rallied her 60 million followers to join us in our fight to protect America's iconic horses.

At every step of this process, Bek and I are meeting with key legislators explaining all the benefits of saving horses: saving veterans from suicide, keeping communities safe by reducing recidivism rates by 50 percent, and saving these beautiful healers from this savage and horrendous slaughter.

Fueled by a purpose and mission like no other, we believed in WHO WE ARE as human beings and our ability to make change in the world, and it has led us to make history. We will not stop until the bill is passed, and our American horses are set free!

How did we get so passionate about horses when had only had them in our lives for such a short period of time?

Here is the story of how we got started:

In 2015, my wife and I took a trip to Los Olivos, California. Every morning I would start the day with a walk with the dogs. We would walk about twenty minutes out along tree-lined streets and quiet roads with nothing but the sound of birds chirping and wind blowing through the trees.

Our turnaround point was at this quaint little farm where there were three horses each in a separate pasture. The horse in the very last pasture would come over to say good morning, every single morning. I would feed her grass over the fence, and she would rub her head up against me and get me to scratch her ears.

She was the most beautiful thing, peaceful, calm, and totally trusting of me. Every morning, I would take the dogs to see Gisele.

Every morning, our bond grew deeper, and every morning her waistline grew a bit wider from my grass feeding.

On the last day of our one-month stay in Los Olivos, I went to say goodbye to Gisele. My heart ached. I would never forget this unexplainable bond that we had created so effortlessly.

Bek and I packed up the car and began our journey home to Colorado. We were passing the local horse store when I yelled out, "Stop! I have one thing I need to do." I hadn't consciously prepared for this to happen; something just made me stop and go in that store. As if sleepwalking, I went in, tried on a cowboy hat, took it up to the counter, and paid. I walked out proudly with the hat on my head. Bek saw me and yelled out, "Why in the world did you buy that? You look ridiculous." I replied almost automatically, "I am manifesting having a horse one day!"

Just like my statement about wanting to become "the best in the world in triathlon," I had made this grand statement not even knowing where it came from. But it came out of my mouth and forever changed my life.

A month later, we were home in Boulder, Colorado when my mom came by with a coupon advertising the Colorado Horse Rescue.

I went in and asked if I could meet some of the horses. The trainer there, Sarah, came out and was nice enough to show me around and educate me more on the fate of so many horses in our country. These chosen few were the lucky ones, being given another chance at a peaceful home and loving life.

I said I wanted to adopt one, and her first questions made my ignorance blatantly obvious.

Do you know how to ride? Have you ever had a horse? Do you have space to keep a horse?

My answers: No, I don't know how to ride. I have never owned a horse, and I live on one acre in Boulder.

"I can change all of this," I said. "I will start taking lessons tomorrow. I will make space on our one acre for a small barn, and I will do whatever it takes to learn what I need to learn to be able to provide a horse with the best possible home and life."

I drove home, signed up for four lessons a week at a local riding school, started cutting down the trees and bushes on our property, and looked up plans for a barn.

I hadn't even adopted a horse yet!

Sarah told me to look at all the horses online and pick one that I would be interested in.

I picked Calypso, an old mare, docile, and very pretty. She reminded me of Gisele.

I went out to the rescue the next day to meet her. Sarah seemed adamant about introducing me to a different horse instead, a sixteen-hand, athletic, six-year-old mare that seemed to be the queen of the rescue. She was ordering everyone else around and clearly was first in line for food, water, attention—and adoption!

I said, "What about Calypso?"

Sarah replied, "She is a bit older, and I just don't think she will be enough for you."

"But I really like her, and I don't even know how to ride…yet."

"Trust me," Sarah said, "Savannah is the *perfect* horse for you. Together you can have an incredible future. You can grow together."

Easily swayed, I thought she must know what she was talking about, so I went in and signed an adoption application, not realizing that this was a formal document saying I was committed to adopting this horse.

I would go by and visit her every day before taking lessons at the riding school. Savannah was one of the most beautiful creatures I had ever seen. You could see every muscle in her body. She was strong and fit, with a presence that was so full of confidence, intensity, and courage. She had a playful side too, but that didn't come out very often, yet...

One day Sarah asked, "Do you want to see her move?"

I said, "Of course I do!"

Sarah had me walk out Savannah to this big sand arena. I was so excited to see her move. Now that I had taken about eight lessons and could now trot on a horse, I felt ready to experience what she might feel like when I finally would get to ride her.

I walked her into the arena and let her loose.

Like a raging bull out of the gate, she took off at a million miles an hour, kicking her back legs into the air and farting at the same time. I had never seen any creature run so fast, so strong, and with so much passion, all while farting explosively.

I was at a loss for words, overcome with her beauty but absolutely terrified at this BEAST that seemed more powerful than a locomotive.

"How would I ever be able to ride that?!"

I was terrified, wondering how in the world I got to this point.

More lessons. More reading. Maybe some hypnosis to overcome my fear of heights and going too fast.

Oh my gosh. It was happening.

I must find a way!

Fast forward two months, and it was time to take Savannah home.

It was time to ride her for the first time. Time to up my lessons and really make a go at being the kind of leader Savannah needed.

Sarah obviously saw something in me that I didn't realize myself. I had to back myself, trust myself, and believe that somehow, someway I could manage this beast and get her to see ME as the one in charge.

Step by step, lesson by lesson, I built up my confidence, finally getting to ride her and eventually going with Sarah out onto the open trails.

I was terrified every time but did it anyway: courage. I showed up as confident and present as I was capable. Horses can read your energy, and if they sense you are insecure, afraid, or under confident, they will take charge and that is never safe for the rider.

I faked it till I made it, and we started forming the most incredible connection.

Sarah decided after five months that it was the right time to take on a fifty-mile endurance ride—kind of like a marathon with horses.

I was absolutely filled with fear and anxiety at the thought of this but didn't want to show Sarah my weakness as she might have found me unfit to be Savannah's owner. So, I said yes.

We went off to Lake George, Colorado to take on this two-day, fifty-mile ride. I didn't just have to successfully ride my horse over obstacles and all different types of terrain—hills, forests, river crossings, and the like—but I also had to manage her excitement being around one hundred other horses tackling the same course, at the same time!

OMG! What am I doing?

I was stretching myself.

I was coming out of my comfort zone, which I hadn't done for a very peaceful two years of my life.

It was time. Time to grow. Time to face my fears. Time to stretch myself by taking on something that seemed impossible.

As I have always done in my life, I was terrified, but I did it anyway.

If you can't, you MUST!

It was the most incredible experience.

In every situation, I was facing something new. I was faced with making decisions constantly and figuring out a way to calm myself, which would calm my horse and lead to our safe arrival at the finish line.

With each challenge, I grew in confidence and trust in my horse.

Savannah was amazing. She and I were discovering ourselves, individually and as a team. Our bond was strengthening and our connection deepening.

She taught me so much along the ride and along the entire journey, showing me what powerful teachers horses are and how sensitive they are to energy.

They are mirrors for us. They will mirror your energy. They will teach you the best possible ways to carry yourself in life to get the responses you are looking for from all those around you.

They teach self-awareness, self-control, boundary setting, resilience, and empathy.

They take you to your deepest truth.

They help you discover all of who you are, what drives you, and what you need so you can grow into the best version of yourself.

She was my teacher.

She had come into my life. I was the student. I was ready. And I didn't even know it.

I was so blown away by the impact Savannah had on me and my life in such a short period of time. One day, I got curious. What did I need to save her from?

I got online and Googled why I would need to rescue a horse. This horrible video came on, showing about sixty horses getting onto a stock trailer meant for cattle. They were crushed on top of each other with no food, no water for a three-to-five-day trip. Many get off the truck with eyes hanging out of their sockets, broken legs, or even dead.

Once they arrived, they were corralled into the slaughterhouse by people hitting their backs with what looked like steel pipes. The screaming. The terror. The devastation. Once in the slaughterhouse, they were taken one by one. They took a captive bolt to the head which 85 percent of the time does

NOT kill them. They then tie up the horses' back legs and pull them up on a pulley, hanging upside down.

At this point, the savages then took a machete to the horses' spines and proceeded to dismember them alive. Blood everywhere. Screaming. All the other horses in line witnessed their family members and friends being dismembered alive, knowing they were next. I have never ever seen anything so horrific.

I fell to the ground in my office wailing, devasted over what I had just seen. My wife came running up the stairs thinking someone had died. I just pointed to the screen as she watched the video. Breaking down in tears and shaking, we looked at each other, and we knew that our lives would never be the same again. We HAD to do something to save these beautiful beings.

No child of God should ever be treated in this way. Horses are healers. They are teachers. They are companions and friends. We have fought wars on their backs. They carried us across the frontiers and have been our partners, friends, and companions for centuries.

These were former lesson horses. These were former racehorses that had made millions of dollars for their owners or a child's best friend, and they were being given up and discarded like trash.

The next day we formed Believe Ranch and Rescue, our nonprofit horse rescue. We saved two horses that first week, and five soon after. Since then, we have saved 195 horses from slaughter, many of whom have gone on to heal humans through equine therapy.

It had come full circle.

Did we dream of doing this? NO! It wasn't even on our radar.

Were we called to do this? Yes, with all our souls. We saw that this must be our mission.

Life happens FOR you, not to you! Do you ever find yourself saying you are going to do something, but you don't know where those words are coming from? Go with it. This is your destiny speaking. You are being called to action. Your purpose is being revealed. Trust in that, find strength in that, and lead with that.

To have the privilege to be more, give more, and create more for others—animals and humans alike—is the most incredible privilege in the world. Go all IN! Don't be afraid, just believe, and be BRAVE!

When I was in the hospital after my bone marrow transplant, there were many times I wondered if I could really survive this. It made me think about my life thus far. Would I be satisfied with how I lived my life to this point?

Three questions came to my mind that I wanted to answer:

> Did I live fully?
> Did I love with all my heart?
> Did I make a difference in this world while I was here?

It became clear to me that those three things were what mattered most to me.

Given the chance to continue to live this miracle of life, I vowed to live every moment in a way that would lead me to answer all three questions in the affirmative at the end of my days.

Those three questions have since guided me to live every moment of my life with purpose, in alignment with what matters most to me.

All I must do is answer the questions: Is this me living fully? Am I loving with all my heart? Will this make a difference somehow in someone else's life? If the answer was yes to all three, I do that thing. If the answer is no, I pass.

I have my compass, and it leads to living life on purpose. I have never felt so fulfilled in my entire life.

I want the same for you.

Remember this:

- If you can't, you MUST!!

- Follow your intuition. This is your soul whispering to you.

- What three questions will matter most to you at the end of your days? Live with the intention of creating those things!

ASSIGNMENT: LEGACY, MISSION, AND PURPOSE

In identifying our purpose or mission, we must first know what matters most to us in our lives.

By prioritizing our top values in previous exercises, we now know the answer to that.

The question becomes "are we living in alignment with those values?"

One way to help you figure out what your purpose or mission is in life is to answer the following questions:

What lights you up? Fills you with energy? Inspires you every day?

1.

2.

3.

4.

5.

How do you want to be remembered?

What is the legacy you most want to leave for others?

How would you most like to hear people eulogize you at your funeral?

What is worth dying for?

What makes your life worth living?

Who do you need to become to achieve this purpose?

What must you let go of?

What must you stop doing?

What must you start doing?

What must you continue to do?

What values must you live by?

1.

2.

3.

What would be three things you would like to teach as many people as possible during this lifetime?

1.

2.

3.

What matters most to you for the rest of this lifetime?

What things can you do to fulfill that desire in the coming day?

In the coming weeks?

In the coming months?

In the coming years?

In the coming decades?

What three questions will you ask yourself at the end of your time here on earth?

1.

2.

3.

At the end of your days, how will you answer this question?

WHO WERE YOU IN THIS LIFETIME?

Chapter 10

THE POWER OF
FORGIVENESS

When I got diagnosed, one of the first things I knew
I had to do was to release any anger, resentment,
or unresolved feelings from my body, sweeping out any tension to make room for the healing to move
through me.

I thought of every person that may have hurt or disappointed me, and I worked through those feelings and emotions. I tried to look at those situations from a different perspective and put myself in their shoes to find compassion.

It was also important to find appreciation for that person
and what happened.

How am I different because of that person? What did I
learn from them? What good came out of that situation?

I needed to also share that same compassion and understanding with myself. I had to let myself off the hook for
not being my best self in that situation and forgive myself
for escalating the drama or making decisions that only made
things worse.

I did the best that I could with the information I had at the time. I did the best that I could with the tools I had to cope at the time.

The people that hurt me were doing the best they could with the information they had at the time and the tools they had available.

The key is that once you know better, you choose to do better.

In 2017, I went to a Tony Robbins Date with Destiny event in Boca Raton, Florida.

This event, from the first five minutes, blew me away. I was amazed by Tony's insights, awareness, and ability to make every person in that room of thousands feel seen, heard, and understood.

On day one, Tony started talking about forgiving the people that have hurt us badly. He spoke of the tremendous burden it was to carry the pain and anger throughout your entire lifetime. This holds us back from living our best lives and finding the joy and fulfillment that we desire.

Tony said, "If you are going to blame that person for all the bad in your life, you also have to blame them for the good."

Sitting there, in a flood of tears, it dawned on me. I had to look at my life since that devastating day. I had become someone that I was so proud of. I had the courage to take on an impossible dream. I found a way to redefine success and failure so that I could always feel as though I was making progress and thus never gave up hope that one day that dream would come true.

I had this insatiable hunger to do whatever it took to one day become a world champion in triathlon.

WHY? Because my father's rejection left me feeling DESPERATE to prove, most importantly, to myself that I mattered, I was worthy, and that I could be loved, by myself and others.

In this desperation, I took risks I never would have before: risks of humiliating myself and risks of massive failure.

Here I had this IVY LEAGUE education from Brown University and the first thing I do with that is chase a dream of being the best at a sport I sucked at.

What would people think? Would I be seen as just throwing this incredible education away? Throwing my life away? Would I be seen as a failure? I didn't care.

My opinion of myself and my trust in myself was that I was a person of substance—a person I could rely on to get me through the toughest storms in life—that mattered much more.

My dad's rejection was a gift!

He was exactly the father I needed him to be so I could become the woman I am so proud to be today.

I ran out of the room, sat on the curb outside the convention center, and cried my eyes out.

I was suddenly seeing everything with a different set of eyes.

Out of the blue, I start remembering the number of times he did call me.

It had been two years without a phone call, so when he first reached out, it gave me the opportunity to let the raging bull of anger off my chest, and I unleashed it all on him.

I called him horrible names and spewed hurt and anger at him.

He tried calling again and again, but this is what I met him with.

Eventually, the calls stopped.

Would you want to call me if that was what you were met with every single time?

No.

Why would you put yourself through that?

All this time, I had conveniently forgotten about those calls. I was so obsessed with my pain and hurt, and I had to blame him for being the worst father ever.

More tears. Now tears of shame. Tears of anger at myself for rejecting him.

It was a crime that equaled his, I realized in that moment. I had to forgive myself first.

At the time, I didn't have the tools that I have now. I didn't know how to manage this tsunami of anger and pain I felt. His call was the trigger that set it all off. This was all I knew, and I didn't know how to move away from these feelings to reach acceptance and appreciation. Until now.

Tony had given me the ultimate gift of perspective.

My father grew up in a family that was very prejudiced, bigoted, racist, and homophobic.

This was ALL HE KNEW.

We often become our parents, adopting their beliefs and responding to life according to them.

At that time, all he knew was what his family had taught him. Gay people will never be accepted. They should be ashamed and locked away, out of sight and not seen in the world.

And then his daughter, who he was so proud of, suddenly dropped this bombshell that she was everything his parents told him was unacceptable.

He did the best that he could with the information he had at the time.

I picked up the phone, and I called my father.

He answered on the first ring! My heart was beating so fast I could barely breathe.

I said, "Dad, you absolutely broke my heart twenty-five years ago when you shunned me when you found out I was gay. But I forgive you and I want to thank you for being exactly the father I needed you to be to become the woman I am so proud to be today."

He started crying and said how sorry he was. He had suffered so much over the years because of what had happened. He told me how proud he was of all that I had achieved and that he loved me.

I had my father back. Forgiveness was the key.

You see, now that he knows better, he does better. Now that I know better, I can do better.

We all make mistakes. But we all have this tremendous ability to change for the better.

Change our beliefs. Change our perspectives.

When we blame others for our pain, or our lack of success, this only hurts us.

It gives you an excuse as to why you didn't take on something you dreamed of. Why you never found that deep, loving relationship. Why you haven't had the success you so deserved.

Remove the shackles and free yourself from the prison of disempowerment and pain that is blame.

Forgiveness is for you!

Forgiveness sets you free.

Forgiveness is you taking your power back.

A beautiful example of the power of forgiveness are the horses we save from the road to slaughter. Most of these horses have been treated horrifically by their previous owners. They are neglected, often abused, or discarded after a lifetime of service once their joints get a bit tight and they can't do the job as they once did.

They come to us terrified. Often their spirit has been broken along with their hearts.

Once they arrive, we shower them with love, patience, and compassion.

We offer them certainty by feeding them at the same times every day. We make sure they have a full trough of water and shelter and a herd to keep them safe. We give them the medical care they need. We speak to them with love and kindness and with a gentleness of words and touch.

Throughout the first two weeks, you see their eyes soften. Their heads relax. They get curious about who we are, and they start opening themselves up to our love and connection.

Within these first few weeks, they forgive humans.

They open themselves up to love and connection and a future of joy and fulfillment.

We don't do this.

As humans, we often hold on to pain and resentment for a lifetime.

This closes us off to all the love and joy we could be experiencing.

These horses are the ultimate example of the power of forgiveness.

We witness them going from broken to strong in body and spirit, from sadness to joy.

Surviving to thriving is so inspiring. It's an example that we all must follow.

Every challenge that I have faced has led me to who I am today.

These challenges, like the one with my father, have led to me become more, so I can give more and create more in my life.

Forgiveness doesn't condone the behavior of the other person. But it means releasing the pain for you and understanding that what is done is done.

You can try to better understand the offender. What must have happened in their life to do what they did to you? Can you find compassion for them? For the circumstances that led them to make the decision they did?

I guarantee you that the person is feeling their own pain over what happened.

Who are you because of what happened?

Think about your greatest qualities, the qualities that have seen you persevere—the qualities that have led to your success in your career or relationships.

Would you have this great strength if what happened had never happened?

Who wouldn't you be had that person not impacted your life in the way they did?

If you are going to blame that person for all the bad, you must also blame them for all the good.

Focusing on the good strengthens and empowers you.

It gives you a new way to look at what happened.

Not forgiving doesn't give you power. It drains you of it.

Not forgiving requires you to carry the burden of pain and resentment along with you wherever you go. It adds a heaviness that holds you back from living life to the fullest.

Once we forgive, we are loving ourselves enough to let go of shame—the shame we often carry due to being a victim of some great offense. It's shame that comes with somehow blaming ourselves for what happened to make sense of it all.

This shame eats away at us, leaving us feeling less than or undeserving of good things in life.

Shame is the birthplace of things like perfectionism. I can attest to this.

Perfectionism hampers success, brings us down, lowers our energy, and leads to us being depressed, anxious, unsatisfied, and full of regret for missed opportunities.

You may think that perfectionism is you striving to be your best, but it is not.

Instead, it is a shield we use to protect ourselves from shame, judgment, and blame.

Aiming to be perfect only leads to more pain, more shame, more judgment, and more blame. It's a vicious cycle that holds us back from all that we want.

We must release the culprit: shame.

It robs us of the joy and fulfillment we yearn for.

The only way to get rid of shame is to practice self-compassion.

FORGIVING yourself is a huge part of this process.

Forgiving OTHERS is a huge part of this process.

Liberate yourself so you can truly live to your fullest potential.

Once we become more loving of ourselves, we can then accept and embrace our own imperfections and begin living truly authentically. To better love ourselves, the first step is forgiveness.

As I was fighting leukemia and sweeping out my soul of any uneasiness that could have caused it, I realized forgiving myself was going to be a huge part of the process.

Every day, being faced with my mortality, I came to love and appreciate myself more and more deeply.

Part of my strategy, which I needed to discipline myself to do in every moment, was stacking my proof. I had proof of the times I had overcome things that seemed impossible, like certain training sessions that had brought me to my knees, relationships that had ripped me apart from the inside out, and overcoming fears that had at one time paralyzed me.

In doing this, I started feeling this deep appreciation for who I was as a human being: my courage, bravery, deep love for others and for life, and burning desire to serve the planet and make a difference for as many lives as I could.

Stacking my proof to survive was also the exercise that led me to deepen my love for myself and gain an appreciation for all that I am.

In this, I started feeling such pain over the DEAL I had made with myself twenty-eight years ago: if I could WIN A WORLD CHAMPIONSHIP, I could love myself.

WHAT? I had to DO something that seemed impossible to give myself permission to love myself?

How cruel and unfair was that? To me?

My heart aches thinking about how high my expectations were for myself, this belief that it would take something extraordinary to earn my own love.

I needed to forgive myself for this. In forgiving myself, I also made a promise that I would always see myself for all that I am—not what I achieve or the things that I "do," but for the "being" that I am:

My passion for life and love.

My gratitude and appreciation for all the grace that surrounds us all.

My desire to want to contribute to the lives around me and make a difference in this world.

In every moment, I see myself and I appreciate myself and I LOVE MYSELF.

Now that I know better, I will do better.

Guilt is born out of an action we took that we feel remorse over. It drives through us when we believe we have caused harm or breached our moral code.

Guilt is often the birthplace of shame, anxiety, depression, and fatigue and can take a devastating toll on one's well-being.

Guilt is typically triggered by something much more minor than the extreme emotional consequences it provokes.

When you are feeling guilty, I encourage you to pause and truly reflect on what you are feeling guilty for from a calm and rational space. When you do this, I am certain you will find that you don't deserve to feel as badly as you do.

Again, I like to direct you to imagine your loved one doing the same thing that you are feeling guilty for. How would you feel about what they have done?

Would it warrant the same punishment that you are giving yourself?

You deserve to have the same compassion, understanding, and love for yourself that you offer all those around you.

Ten years ago, my incredible mom lost her soulmate doggie, Buddha.

I always say that when I die, I want to come back as one of my mom's pugs.

She treats them as if they are her children, feeding them better than she feeds herself.

They get kibble with some salmon, turkey, green beans, and cottage cheese every single night. And they finish it off with a spoonful of peanut butter for dessert. Then, my mom eats.

She hikes with them every day and lets them take up the whole bed at night. She sleeps one leg off the side, squeezed in the corner, as her three pugs sprawl out across the queen-sized bed.

Buddha was having some horrible knee pain and was not enjoying the hikes anymore.

My mom took him to several doctors, all of whom said the only way to figure out what was going on was to do an MRI.

She took their advice and scheduled the MRI.

Buddha went in for this common procedure and never came out.

They had given him too much fentanyl that led to brain damage and a quick death.

My mom was brokenhearted, ravaged by the loss of her precious soulmate.

She blamed herself. She kept saying how she killed him. It was all her fault.

How could she have done this to her own child?

The pain of losing Buddha was now overshadowed by the pain she felt within herself.

The guilt. The anger.

She tortured herself not just for days, weeks, or months but for years.

She would start crying a week out from the anniversary of his death, spewing words of anger toward herself for killing him. It was so painful to witness this.

I kept saying, "You didn't know this was going to happen! You were doing what you thought was the right thing for him. Get an MRI, treat whatever the problem was, and get him back to the glorious walks that you both cherished every day."

She didn't know what she knows now! If she had known that this was going to happen, she would have never taken him in there.

Finally, she realized that she truly did do what she thought was right at the time.

She couldn't have imagined that Buddha would die from an MRI.

She chose to free herself from the blame and accept what had happened as just a horrible, sad fate that Buddha met on that day. I had her focus on the amazing mom she had been for him and all her pugs, stacking her proof of that every time she started feeling guilt.

Finally, in forgiving herself and releasing the blame, she opened herself up to being the best pug mom once again. She rescued her new boy Buddha in September of 2021 and has given herself permission to receive his love and to welcome the joy and fulfillment that he brings her.

Can you relate to this story?

Can you look back at some decisions you made that didn't work out the way you had hoped?

Did you know then what you know now?

Forgive yourself. Appreciate where you are now and open yourself up to all the freedom and love you deserve.

Forgiveness is a gift you give yourself.

Letting go is your ticket to freedom.

Letting go frees you to write a new story in life that is more aligned with your purpose and mission.

It's a new story that sets you free—free to live the life that you dream of and inspiring all those around you to do the same.

Remember this:

- Forgiveness is for YOU!

- Forgive yourself and forgive others so that you can liberate yourself to truly live life to your fullest potential.

- Now that you know better, do better.

- Remove the shackles and free yourself from the prison of disempowerment and pain that is blame.

ASSIGNMENT: FORGIVENESS EXERCISE

FORGIVENESS

Who in your life have you been unable to forgive for the pain inflicted upon you (whether physical, emotional, or mental pain)?

What is your belief around what happened?

Because of this _____ I am,
I don't have, or I have _____

What if the opposite was true?

For example: My dad was never home. He didn't love us.
He didn't want to be with us. We never saw him and didn't
have any kind of relationship because of that.

What if he was working so many hours because he loved
you so much and wanted to make sure he could provide for
you and give you everything you needed?

If you are going to blame this person for the bad, you must
also blame them for the good.

Can you think of aspects of your life that would not be what they are had this not happened?

1.

2.

3.

Who would you NOT be if this hadn't happened?

1.

2.

3.

Who wouldn't be in your life if this hadn't happen?

1.

2.

3.

What wouldn't you know if this hadn't happened?

1.

2.

3.

To truly free yourself to be open to LOVE, SUCCESS, JOY, and FULFILLMENT, you must find it within yourself to forgive and even thank this person for being exactly who you needed them to be so you could become the amazing human you are today.

Think about what you could say to this person and write below:

How do you think this would make you feel to follow through in forgiving them (either by phone, by email, or just energetically inside yourself)?

What would you be free of if you did this?

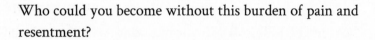
Who could you become without this burden of pain and resentment?

Time to Forgive Yourself

What must you forgive yourself for?

Why must you forgive yourself?

Did you know then what you know now?

If you didn't know then what you know now, can you have compassion for yourself?

What are the consequences of not forgiving yourself?

What are the consequences for the people you love and care about?

How can you look at what happened, or didn't happen, with a different perspective?

If your most beloved did the same thing that you have not forgiven yourself for, what would you say to them? Would you forgive them for it? Why?

Can you show that same compassion for yourself? Why is this important?

What good will come out of you forgiving yourself? How will you be different?

Now that you know better, you will do better! That is what matters most!

Give yourself grace and love yourself enough to set yourself free.

Chapter 11

THE POWER OF THE UNEXPECTED TEACHER

One of the most important missions I have been on my whole life has been wanting to know myself. To come home to my truth.

There is a beautiful quote usually attributed to Michelangelo:

> "I saw the angel in the marble, and I carved until I set her free."

My whole life has been about chipping away at the marble that has been my disempowering stories, self-doubt, fears, and anxieties with the ultimate hope of revealing my angel. It is my authentic self, minus all the stuff that isn't me—the thoughts and beliefs that were luring me away from my true self.

Every great goal I have taken on has been with that mission in mind.

I want you to find this as well. UNBECOME the parts of you that aren't the real you and come home to your truth, with all the beauty and magic of who you are.

One of the most powerful ways I have done this has involved animals.

They have been some of my greatest sources of love my entire life and some of my most powerful teachers.

"When the student is ready, the teacher appears."

The whole story I shared earlier of horses coming into my life is a perfect example of that.

Savannah was that teacher for me.

I never would have believed that one day I would have horses.

In 2007, my soulmate cat Gertie died of cancer. I had tried for months to keep her alive through exploratory treatments at the Colorado State University Veterinary Teaching Hospital. I drove her back and forth multiple times a week, but it wasn't meant to be. My dear girl passed, and I was devastated.

I called an animal communicator as I was so desperate to somehow stay connected to my beloved cat.

She said to me, "Gertie needs to rest but she will come back in some years to live another lifetime with you. She will come back as a horse."

I was so upset, thinking, "This woman has no idea what she is talking about."

Why would I ever have a horse?

Nine years later and destiny would have it that Savannah came into my life.

Wow. To this day, this awes me.

Savannah would prove to be exactly what I needed in my life at that time, and her teachings would give me everything I needed to tackle AML.

Horses see you for exactly who you are.

We often don't see ourselves that way.

We believe the stories we have told ourselves about our imperfections—the stories we tell ourselves about our worth and our lovability.

Horses see YOU. The truth about you: your essence, your spirit, your heart, and your soul.

They meet you where you are at any given moment.

Watch the dynamics of a horse herd and you will see that horses embody tolerance, non-judgment, compassion, patience, forgiveness, and unconditional acceptance.

Imagine if we not only treated all those around us in this way, but even more importantly, if we treated ourselves with this same kind of acceptance, love, and non-judgment.

Imagine if you always stood in the truth of your higher self.

Imagine knowing your heart. Knowing how deep you love. How good your intention is. How much you care and how hard you try. Imagine having that be enough for you to love, honor, and value yourself in every moment.

When we as humans emulate these traits of the horse, we grow and expand. We get one step closer to coming home to our authentic truth. That centeredness and grounded-ness bring us peace and calm.

Horses can see your truth. They know exactly what you are feeling. They don't judge you or your behaviors. They accept you unconditionally.

Horses mirror back the exact same feelings, attitudes, and intentions that you are feeling.

Their mirroring is through non-verbal behavior. It is through their body language that they will express their feelings.

For example, if a horse thinks that your intention will feel good, it will stay around you. If they don't, they will walk away and avoid you.

As humans, we all can agree that it feels good when people do things for us. But it's not so good when people do things TO us.

If you want a horse to come to you and they don't, the problem is not the horses. Often, we will want the horse to change and come to us. We do this in life as well. We want to change the people around us, change their behavior, or change their feelings. This isn't possible. The question is: What do you need to change?

You are the one that must change to get a different response.

What can you do differently?

What must change in your actions, energy, or intention to develop a relationship with the horse?

The same thing goes in life. We must focus on what we can control, not on what we can't.

You CANNOT change another person. You cannot control how they respond and react to you, or to life.

You DO, however, have control over how you respond and react to life. You can control what you focus on and how you feel in any given moment.

To develop a relationship with a horse, you must develop a keener sense of self and recognize how your actions impact others.

Horses will provide you with these insights during your interactions with them.

Horses have three things that matter most to them in life:

1. Survival: not being eaten
2. Comfort: food, water, and avoiding pain
3. Position in the herd: knowing who is in charge will ensure that the above two things are being taken care of

Considering a horse's top values, you can better understand how to develop a meaningful relationship with them. Keep them safe. Provide them with their basic needs and do things FOR them or with them, not to them.

To develop a meaningful relationship with a horse, you must prove yourself as a leader. You must be someone they can trust and rely on. They can trust you to keep them safe, lead with fairness and consistency, and bring them comfort, not pain.

Forming a relationship with a horse guides you to your own self-awareness.

What do you need most in life? In the last section, you uncovered your top values. What are your top three values?

In seeing how important those things are for you, you can understand and relate to how important the horse's top values are to them.

While developing a relationship with Savannah, I learned so much about myself: how expectations often derail me and leave me discouraged, how I needed to become more patient, and how I needed to embrace the process, not impatiently push for an outcome.

It reinforced how important resilience is.

When something isn't working, don't just give up and move on to something different.

You must stay on the path. What can you learn from your mistakes or disappointments?

How can you change your approach to get a different result?

In learning to ride Savannah, I was so eager to go from not being able to ride to galloping in a field at sunset. It's kind of like not knowing how to swim but wanting to become a world-champion triathlete.

That certainly didn't happen overnight. It took me eight years to achieve that goal, and it took many failures along the way.

I showed resilience then, so why was I struggling with patience now?

Somehow, I thought that since I was older and wiser, I should be better at this. I should pick it up quicker. But that is not how life works.

Can you think of a time recently when you tried something new and it didn't go so well, so you just quit? What was it that got in the way of you continuing to try? Was it a lack of patience? Or an unwillingness to fail?

Anything new takes us back to learning how to walk or how to ride a bike. No matter how old or mature we are, we still must start from square one.

Fall over a few times, feel the insecurity and the fear, but work each day toward getting a tiny bit better.

When a child is learning to walk, he/she will fall over many times before finally walking successfully. WE don't tell them to give up after falling five or six times. We get excited each time they take one more step than the time before.

WE must give ourselves that same kind of support and belief—that soon we will get to where we want to go.

Celebrate each step along the way. Learn from your mistakes and persevere through the uncomfortable moments.

Developing a relationship with Savannah and getting her to trust me involved all these things.

When I finally could ride, it wasn't riding I learned how to do.

I had learned to connect deeply in such a beautiful way that would forever impact my connections with others through non-verbal communication and the importance of energy and self-awareness.

I had built up my resilience that would translate to life.

I had built up my self-awareness that would improve my relationships.

I had built up EMPATHY. Recognizing and relating to Savannah's feelings would allow me to better recognize and understand other people's feelings and situations in relationships.

I learned a lot about self-regulation, which is the KEY to emotional well-being.

I learned to monitor my responses to things that happen to me to better support the outcome.

I adjusted my energy and focus to help me better navigate difficult situations or moments in my life.

As scared as I was, I wanted desperately to ride my beautiful mare. I knew that to do so, I needed to form a bond with her where she trusted me, and I trusted her.

This trust gave me more confidence, not only in myself but more importantly, in our partnership. We were in this together. I understood her, and she understood me. This led to riding her with a confidence my training hadn't quite yet earned me, but the relationship we had developed did.

The whole process of leaning into the unknown and learning all these new things at age forty-seven showed me that I was so much braver than I believed and so much more courageous than I could have imagined.

Think about how all the above gave me such a powerful foundation to live my life. It's such a beautiful gift.

When I am with horses, I am reminded of who I am: the beauty, magic, and love that I am.

For me, nothing compares to the feeling I get when I am with my horses.

A sense of peace and calm.

A KNOWING that I am okay.

This is the place I go to reconnect. To find balance. To get centered and grounded.

Still, it is a place I go to learn, grow, and equip myself to make progress in my life in other ways, every day.

Where in your life are you taught similar lessons? Where in your life do you go to find your center? To learn and to grow?

How much have you learned from your kids or your animals?

We learn loyalty and find joy in the simple pleasures of life from our pets.

Dogs, horses, and children teach us how to live in the now and how to forgive and forget.

Children teach us unbridled joy.

Maybe you find your growth, learning, and center in reading books or listening to music. What is your preferred mode of learning?

I have found music to be a loyal friend throughout my entire life.

It's been a teacher in so many ways.

When I first realized I was gay, I had so many questions that I didn't have the answer to.

I would listen endlessly to music by Melissa Etheridge. Her album *Yes I Am*, released in 1993, was believed to be her coming-out album.

Melissa is a two-time Grammy winner and an Academy Award winner for her song "I Need to Wake Up" from *An Inconvenient Truth*.

Her words made me feel seen and understood while I was isolated and alone in my self-inflicted closet.

Many years later, twenty-six to be exact, I had the privilege of meeting the rock legend herself, Melissa Etheridge, and her amazing wife, Linda Wallem. From the moment we met, we knew this would be the beginning of a lifelong friendship.

Melissa and Linda are two of the most down-to-earth humans I have ever met.

Melissa has this deep wisdom that I experienced through her music in my twenties. She was a teacher to me then and continues to be now. Throughout my battle with AML,

Melissa and Linda were there for Bek and me not only as loving friends but as teachers helping us navigate this foreign and terrifying territory that was cancer.

Think about this: You are a mentor to the people who witness you living your life. Whether you know it or not, you are teaching the people around you. Tony Robbins always asks, "Are you an example or a warning?"

Think about the unexpected teachers in your life. Have they shown you what to do? Or what not to do? Who have you learned from? What have you learned from?

Pay attention. Be present. These are beautiful gifts that can transform the world and how you see yourself.

What can you do to grow today and in the future?

As a coach, I have always demanded of myself the same growth and learning that I ask of my athletes. If I am asking them to grow and expand their abilities every single day, then I must do the same.

As a leader, we must be examples of what we ask for in others.

This becomes a constant motivator for the people you lead, whether that be your family, your herd, your team, or your organization.

Remember:

- Be present to what you can learn from your mistakes or disappointments. When we fail, we learn, and when we learn, we grow. This is HOW we make progress.

- Be present to what you can learn from people, animals, nature, books, and music.

- Go first in being what you hope to see in others.

ASSIGNMENT: RECOGNIZING YOUR TEACHERS

What can you do today to initiate growth in some area of your life?

What will you do tomorrow?

What can you stop doing that gets in the way of your growth or learning?

What will you do more of?

How will this help you in your life?

List three people you have learned from in your lifetime.

1.

2.

3.

What were your most powerful learnings from each?

1.

2.

3.

Is there an animal, being, or species that has taught you a valuable life lesson?
What was it?
What did you learn?

In the last ninety days what did you learn?

1.

2.

3.

4.

5.

Who were the people you learned from and inspired you?

     1.

     2.

     3.

     4.

     5.

What did you learn about yourself in the last ninety days?

     1.

     2.

     3.

     4.

     5.

What species or group can you observe and learn from?

Who can you observe that you can learn from?

Chapter 12

THE POWER
OF DECISIONS

One of my favorite book series I loved to read as a kid was the Choose Your Own Adventure books.

These books gave me hope. Hope that with certain decisions, life could get better and that we all weren't stuck going in one direction, feeling the same feelings repeatedly. Things could change for the better.

I would read these books and go on adventures in my mind. I got to choose. No one else.

I got to choose my own adventure and that felt so good to me.

During this time, I felt so out of control. I was bound to the grip of my fear of needing to be a rock for everyone else around me. I was a rock that was hollow on the inside, like those fake rocks you hide your keys in and leave by the side of your front door.

(Yep, now you can all enter my house at any point, hehe.)

The Choose Your Own Adventure books inspired me to one day make decisions according to what I wanted. They would be decisions that felt like the right decision for ME.

Ultimately, when I was at Brown, I had the epiphany that ONLY I have the power to change my experience of life. I took all that I had learned from those books and decided what adventure my new life would start with.

That led to Club Med, and that led to playing ice hockey after being prohibited from doing so by my field hockey and lacrosse coach. It led to me experimenting with my sexuality.

The Choose Your Own Adventure books showed us all that decisions matter. They truly do shape your destiny. For that reason, the power of decisions is a very important member of the Power Line.

Decisions must be made with some thought. Decisions must reflect what matters most to you.

Now, sometimes your gut is screaming so loud at you to do something. Those decisions made from the gut, I believe, can be made quickly! Trust in that gut feeling that has never led you astray. Trust in the deep pull that is your soul whispering to you. As the pull gets stronger, that whisper becomes louder and something you simply can't ignore.

One example of this: I had been living out in California for six years. A terribly unhealthy relationship lured me out there. I had come to love the place, and frankly, just didn't feel like going through a big move once again.

I started dating my future wife in 2013. We were living together in Santa Monica in a tiny five-hundred-square-foot cottage. This is how I knew I loved her. I usually was not comfortable sharing space with anyone, especially such a tiny space. But together, we gave that adorable cottage a heartbeat. It was cozy. It was comfortable. It became a sanctuary for me. For the first time, I had a sanctuary that I shared with another person. That didn't take away from the sacredness of what "HOME" had always meant to me. Somehow, it felt more like a home sharing it with her.

I went home for a week to visit my mom back in Boulder, Colorado. That was where I lived from 1995 to 2007.

The day before I was meant to drive home, I decided to run on one of my favorite trails out at the Boulder Reservoir.

It felt so good to be running in the fresh mountain air. No traffic, no smog, and such a beautiful view all around me. I was adding to the loop to satisfy my lingering OCD tendencies. I needed to make it an hour flat.

So, I ran down this residential street just off the reservoir trail. At exactly an hour I landed in front of this beautiful blue house eight hundred meters from where I had parked my car. It had a For Sale sign in front of it.

"Wow, what a great area to live in. No need to drive to run around the reservoir, and I could coach my athletes right out my front door."

I pulled the flyer out and called the number.

This house had been on the market for over six months. They had just lowered the price that day, and I was the first to inquire about it.

The price of this house, with 3,500 square feet and two acres of land, sitting eight hundred meters away from my favorite run trail, cost the same as what I had paid for my five-hundred-foot cottage in Santa Monica.

I asked if I could see the place on that day, as I was driving back to LA the next day.

He said the owner typically didn't take walkthroughs on Sundays, but he would see if they could make an exception for me.

An hour later, I was walking through the house. I felt as though it was already mine. I felt like the house wrapped its arms around me the moment I walked through the door.

I just knew. This was meant to be.

I put in an offer that afternoon and the next morning they told me they had accepted it. I was over the moon.

This all happened so fast, I hadn't yet had the chance to tell Bek.

I called her and asked, "Do you like Boulder, Colorado?"

She said, "I've never been there but my identical twin sister Simmy says it's one of her favorite places in the world. Why do you ask?"

"I just bought a house. Will you move to Boulder with me?"

Fortunately, we were early on in our relationship. I justified to myself that we weren't at the point yet where we made big life decisions together.

I fell more in love with Bek the moment she said, "Sure. Why not? Wow."

Within three months, I had sold my place in Santa Monica, and we moved to our amazing new home in Boulder.

This changed EVERYTHING for us. My coaching business grew immediately as every athlete wants to train in Boulder. All the athletes I had been coaching did not LOVE the fact that if I coached them, they had to train in Los Angeles. Although the training was amazing, getting there was the problem. It was hours in traffic to get to the best running and riding roads and trails.

My former athlete Mirinda Carfrae, who lived in Boulder, found the courage to ask if I would coach her again. I was beyond excited to have a chance to finish what we started together. We went on to win two more world championship crowns together.

This never would have happened if I stayed in California.

I achieved so much with my athletes in those first three years back in Colorado that I was feeling pulled to write a book.

My wife and I, to get away somewhere from daily responsibilities, flew to Los Olivos, California for her to train and for me to write my book.

That was when I met Gisele, the horse down the road that I would visit on my daily walks with my dogs.

If I hadn't met Gisele, I wouldn't have heard the whisper of my soul saying, "Horses!"

If I hadn't heard that whisper, I wouldn't be here today living on a ranch with my beautiful wife and horses, having saved 178 beautiful lives from slaughter.

If I hadn't saved Savannah, the FIRST of those 178 horses, I probably would not have done, achieved, and survived what I have over the past five years.

DECISIONS MATTER

Choose your own adventure.

Trust your gut and listen to the whispers of your soul.

DECISIONS SHAPE YOUR DESTINY

Think about decisions such as what school to go to?

Who to spend your life with?

Decisions about your health.

Decisions about what career to follow. Which job to take?

The best decisions are those made in consideration of what you value most in life.

Often decisions are made with a DECLARATION.

Declare, "One day, I am going to be the best in the world in this sport" to your bewildered but ever-supportive mom.

"I am DONE with this job, relationship, thought pattern, disempowering story…"

"Yes, I will marry you!"

The declaration is THE most powerful part of any decision. At that moment, you become accountable to whoever is standing next to you and to God, the universe, or whatever higher power you may believe in.

Moments after being handed my diagnosis, I declared to my bawling wife and my doctor on speaker phone:

"I am going to SURVIVE, and I am going to THRIVE."

In that moment, I laid out the precedent for everyone else to follow.

You must believe, as I do, that we will FIND A WAY to conquer this.

THIS WILL BE MY MOST BEAUTIFUL TRIUMPH. PERIOD.

Every person in my life, every doctor, and every nurse knew that that was my intent and what I was focusing on.

Nothing upset me more than people coming up to me with sad and frightened eyes saying their final goodbyes. Yes, it was sweet and heartfelt and with such good and loving intention. But I am NOT DYING!!

I know I look like I am. I know that is what the statistics would say.

But my spirit is ALIVE, my SOUL wants to live, and I can see myself thriving on the other side of this.

PLEASE see the possibility of that as well. For me. Please.

When we get everyone on board with our vision and our decision, we then create an energy source that is like the wind on your back on a bike ride. That gentle assistance makes everything feel a little bit better and helps you get to where you want to go.

Can you remember the biggest decisions you made in your life? Or a decision that changed your life in a profound way?

Who did you declare it to?

When I made the decision to SURVIVE and THRIVE that meant that every single thought I had, every action I took, and every belief I made mine was with THAT outcome in mind.

If I found myself thinking opposite thoughts, which inevitably I did all the time, I would change the channel.

1. Became aware of this thought and how it made me feel.
2. Asked myself if believing this thought was going to help me heal and get me where I wanted to go: survival and triumph.

3. When the answer came back as a resounding "NO!" I would then change the channel. I constantly redirected my focus from fear to love, from despair to gratitude, from hopelessness to reminding myself of the strength and the proof I have of successfully getting through other great challenges in my life.

4. Stacked my proof in every moment. I reminded myself of the challenges I had overcome—things I had achieved that seemed impossible.

5. Constantly disciplined my mind. I ensured that most of the time I was feeding my mind thoughts that strengthened me and gave me hope and energy.

6. Reframed everything that was happening to me. Chemo was healing me. Thank you. Pneumonia was just my body telling me I was doing too much and needed to slow down. The leukemia was here to teach me something. What I was going through then was preparing me for what I asked for. What would my story of triumph be? What lessons would I be able to share that could save other people's lives? I was writing it all down and being present in every moment to the "possible future gifts" that would come out of this horrendous struggle.

This was a continual process. I needed to consistently question my thoughts and whether they were hurting me or helping me.

This was a DECISION to stand guard at the gates of my mind, turn away the thoughts that would derail me, but invite all those that were crucial to my survival.

I am going to share with you one of the scariest and most painful things that I have ever had to manage in my heart, mind, and spirit.

It was days after receiving my diagnosis, and I needed to figure out HOW I was going to have it treated. What would give me the best chances of survival?

I had so many amazing people wanting to help me. They were giving me amazing advice on hospitals to visit, treatments that were being researched, and other places to go.

I was referred to a naturopath doctor that had a very good reputation.

My gut was already telling me what I KNEW I needed to do. But I was so scared in the moment and was having a harder time trusting my gut feeling that I had always relied on. I couldn't make a mistake!

So, I went to see the doctor and after spending a few hours, he asked me to come to his office to discuss the plan.

I spoke before he could go any further. "I have decided that I am going to go with a clinical trial that has just started at a hospital in Colorado where I live. UCHealth Anschutz has two of the top leukemia doctors in the country. They feel confident in their plan. The clinical trial will put me into remission over a few months. As soon as I get into remission, they will put me in hospital, pound my body with chemo and radiation, wipe out my entire immune system, and right at that point do a life-saving bone marrow transplant. I believe in this. I know in my gut this is the right thing to do. This is what will save my life."

He looked at me with disdain and said, "So, you're doing this to make your family happy?"

I said, "NO, I am doing this for me. I want to live. This decision MUST be mine and mine alone."

He said, "Well, you can start saying your goodbyes because that will never work. You are going to die."

Those words "you are going to die."

Struck me like a knife.

Rattled me to the core.

It infused this enormous amount of doubt that came storming through the gates of my mind, knocking over the guards that were meant to keep things like that out.

Bek grabbed my hand and pulled me out of there so quickly. She held me so tight as I cried.

Terrified. Falling apart.

I had gone from one moment knowing in my heart that the decision I had made was the one that would save my life, confident and certain in sharing it with this man.

Two minutes later, here I was.

Feeling broken in spirit. In heart. Exhausted to my core.

Bek held me and her love poured through her heart into mine.

She had no words. We were both shocked by the man's heartlessness.

When she finally spoke, she said, "This is exactly WHY this is not the man whose hands you put your life in."

We left, got on the next flight home, and sat there shaking, in shock, over what had happened.

I had to regroup. I had to focus on the facts:

I KNEW with absolute certainty that my chosen path was the one that would save my life.

Every decision I had made in the past with that kind of certainty had been the right decision.

Why? Because when you go ALL IN on believing in something, your entire being gets on board. It then will do everything it can to play out the vision you have. You manifest it in your imagination and then your body and soul align with this vision.

But it takes one million percent belief.

It takes making the decision. Not floundering. But ACTING. DECIDING and then never looking back.

Never questioning it.

As Tony Robbins says, "If you want to take the island you have to burn the boats!"

I called Dr. Dan Pollyea, the incredible doctor who had developed the clinical trial. It would involve two drugs, Venetoclax and Azacitidine, and a protocol he created and believed in for me.

I declared to Dr. Pollyea: "I am IN! When can we start?"

I went in the next day, and we got started.

I would be the seventh person in the WORLD to partake in this trial.

I met Dr. Gutman, who was going to be my oncologist. He is a brilliant man who was taken aback initially by my hug, thanking him for saving my life before we even started. He had this silent confidence, this deep wisdom that I trusted in immediately.

The treatment Dr. Gutman would use for me was also a clinical trial.

I met the amazing nurses that would be by my side every step of the way.

The first nurse who met me at the door, Taylor Manns, would become a constant source of comfort for me and a forever friend.

I had my wife, I had my mom, and I was ready.

This was going to be my A-TEAM and today I call them MY DREAM TEAM.

When you decide, pay attention to how that decision feels in your gut.

What do you KNOW inside that is the right thing to do?

There are no wrong decisions.

The decision that you make, that you go ALL IN ON, will be the right decision for you, always.

Listen to your gut.

TRUST in the choice you are making.

Have FAITH that it is THE right thing for you. Not for someone else, but for YOU!

GO ALL IN and never stop believing.

> Remember this:
>
> • The best decisions are those that are made in consideration of what you value most in life.
>
> • There are no wrong decisions.
>
> • The decision that makes you go ALL IN ON will be the right decision for you, always.

ASSIGNMENT: DECISIONS

What do you believe about decisions?

Is this belief serving you? Is it leading you to making good decisions?

What are the consequences of believing this?

What must change?

What can you believe about decisions now?

List three of the biggest decisions you have had to make in your life.

1.

2.

3.

Can you remember the process you took to make that decision?
Describe in detail here:

Think about three bad decisions you have made that didn't work out the way you wanted them to. How can you describe these decisions?

Did you decide in terms of what would be best for another person, not you?

Were you pressured to make that decision?

Was it a SHOULD or a MUST?
Describe in detail:

In making important decisions, what three things can you use as guidelines to set yourself up for success?

Chapter 13

THE POWER OF RESILIENCE

Resilience holds a very strong place on the Power Line. It is required of you on this journey.

What does resilience mean to you?

To me, resilience is as important as the air we breathe.

If you don't get up after you fall, you cut off the blood supply to your future dreams.

If you don't work through your emotions and instead numb them with drinking, drugs, overeating, or losing yourself in work, you blind yourself to all the good.

Joyful moments, grace, and magic moments would give you hope and reason to come out of your pain.

This again cuts off your circulation and keeps you stuck.

If you don't work hard day after day to become better at the things you care about, you will stay the same.

When I coach my athletes, I have them go harder in training than they will ever have to go in a race. Why? Because I want race day to be a CELEBRATION of all the hard work they have done and NOT a test to see if they can do it.

I want them to meet the demons they will face in the toughest moments on the course ahead of time. I want them to KNOW those demons well on race day when they inevitably show up, and my athlete will have plenty of proof of the times they have knocked those demons down.

If my athlete's key race is on a hilly course, we will run and ride hills way harder than the ones they will see on the course. We will ride those hills until they master the feeling of the grind and the push required to climb them confidently.

In riding those hills long and hard in training, they arrive prepared on race day to elevations and descents that they have mastered physically and mentally in their minds. The course they face will have no different requirements from my athlete than those they faced at home. GRIT. GRACE. STRENGTH. CONFIDENCE. RESILIENCE.

There is nothing new my athletes need to ask of themselves on this day.

All they must do is show up and do what they always do.

This practice builds resilience, confidence, strength, and unshakeable mental toughness.

Look at resilience like this: by digging deep through the hard times, taking on BIG CHALLENGES, and going THROUGH the pain leads to an easier future for you, not a harder one.

Staying safe and saving all your best for when the challenge hits only leads to it being much harder to overcome.

Digging deep, busting through limitations, and facing your fears daily will prepare you well for any challenge that comes your way. Suddenly those challenges don't seem so scary or so hard.

The confidence you have built to do those things that make you uncomfortable gives you a greater capability to FIND A WAY through anything.

Resilience is built when we struggle and when we are faced with a deep challenge that really tests our strength, our heart, and our will. It may seem like an impossible situation, where every way you turn you get slapped in the face, but you MUST NOT GIVE UP.

The longer you keep showing up and leaning in, the stronger you become. The more confidence you build. The better prepared you are.

When the challenge arrives, you can roll up your big girl or boy sleeves and face it for all that it is. Allow yourself to experience the feelings and emotions that it carries. Or you can numb it.

If you have been stuck numbing your feelings, it is time to WAKE UP.

Think about everything you want in life.

Notice how you feel now.

Assess what matters most to you.

Are you living life in a way that will get you closer to living in alignment with what matters most to you?

Will it get you all that you want in life?

It is so important to see the quicksand numbing puts you in.

You may feel as though you are succeeding in ignoring the pain, but inside of you a baby monster is growing, and eventually, you must face each other in the ring of life.

Work through your pain. Experience the grief, loss, sadness, or anger that you feel inside. This will give you the strength you need to move beyond it.

It is in the act of facing it that creates an opening for you to strengthen and move beyond it.

I didn't just go to the pool, look at the swim lane, and become a great swimmer.

I had to dive in, despite my fear. I had to find a way to float, find a way to move forward, find a way to ultimately swim lap after lap with energy and force to become the triathlete I dreamed of becoming.

It was imperative that I remembered WHY I was putting myself through this humiliating and often frustrating process.

It mattered enough to me to keep me showing up to the pool day after day.

I was fueled by the goal of being a little bit better, whether that meant less fearful, more proficient, faster, stronger, or fitter. Often, I just wanted to not have to fight it so much. I wanted more flow, not force, and this came from building resilience.

I HAD TO DO THE WORK. There was no way around it.

Your pain is the same way. You can look at it, numb it, and ignore it, but it will be there until you finally duke it out and work your way through it.

Sometimes, you can ignore it, and over time you feel you "lost" the monster.

All it takes is something that triggers that initial pain, and it comes back, sometimes stronger than it was before.

It will come back to haunt you.

I want you to commit to leaving no unfinished business with your pain, anger, resentment, or sadness.

Invite it in for a heart-to-heart conversation.

Get to know it better. This will perhaps give you a different perspective on it, which will lessen its sting.

Resolve to work through it, better understand it, accept it for what it was, and move on.

What can you learn from having communed with your emotions?

Feel the strength your deeper awareness gives you.

When going through this "work," balance it out with doing things that bring you joy. Surround yourself with people that you love. Give them love and be open to receiving it in return.

All the love and joy you feel in life is often born in pain. We cannot have light without darkness. Joy without pain.

Refraining from numbing your pain will give you the incredible capacity to truly embrace the joy that comes on the other side.

If you numb the pain, you also numb the joy.

Resilience is built upon a foundation of continuing when you don't think you can.

Digging deeper when you feel you have nothing left.

Trying again regardless of how many times you fail-ed before.

Reframing each challenge as the beautiful opportunity it is.

Think about babies. When they start crawling, you know that soon, they will try to walk.

When they do, they fall over, hit their head, and cry.

Try again. Fall over again. Hit their elbow and cry, repeatedly.

You don't tell them to just give up at that point, do you?

Why not?

Because you know that if they keep trying and never give up, they will one day be able to walk.

Well, so can you.

Let's go back to that resilient baby version of ourselves and remember that.

We did it then, and we can do it again.

I will never forget my first day at training camp in Switzerland with my coach Brett Sutton.

I was swimming and going as hard as I possibly could.

He came over to the side of the pool and said, "Go harder."

I said, "This is it; this is as hard as I can possibly go."

He said again, "GO HARDER."

There was no sense arguing with him.

As I continued swimming, I kept asking myself, "Can I? Could there possibly be more?"

Of course, there was, but the problem was I had this governor switch that was programmed to go off when I felt a certain overwhelmingly uncomfortable amount of pain.

When the switch went off, I ran out of gears—mental gears, I came to understand, not physical.

It was up to me to break through previous perceived levels of exertion and venture into the unknown.

So, in every session of swimming, biking, and running, I started challenging these perceived limits.

I disconnected my governor switch and instead, slowly but consistently, started building up the amount of time I pushed harder than I thought I could.

It took coaching myself through it by saying, "Okay, you haven't been here before, but we are going there today! If I die, I die, but if I don't, I will reach a whole new level of physical fitness and mental toughness. All of which will get me one step closer to achieving my dream."

So, each day I explored my limits and came to find that every time I did, I survived. It hurt like hell and scared me, but I survived, and I lived to tell the tale.

This is resilience: refusing to give in to perceived limits, refusing to give in when it looks like you have lost the fight, and refusing to give up on a dream that drives you.

Resilience builds character. Character builds champions. Character brings you one step closer to the realization that we truly operate at probably about 60 percent of our capabilities most of the time. Imagine what this means for your own potential!

Resilience can be an attitude. When you give it an empowering meaning, it suddenly becomes an attitude. A badge of honor. I certainly took this on as a major part of my identity.

"She just never gives up."

"She sinks her teeth into something and just will NOT let go."

"Siri is just relentless."

"Don't tell Siri she can't because she WILL."

I was proud of this being part of my identity. I would never give up no matter the circumstances.

If it is something that matters to me, I am willing to get beat up—right, left, and center—and will search out any and every sign of hopefulness, latch onto that, and find a way to victory.

I did it in triathlon.

I did it to triumph over AML.

I am doing it now FOR THE HORSES.

The secret ingredient is resilience.

Just like every baby in the world, keep giving it your all every single day.

Take the falls as learning experiences. As you keep going, you are building resilience and character, resourcefulness and toughness.

All babies know is that they want to walk and will not stop until they figure out how and build up the strength to do it.

Remember this:

- Resilience is built upon a foundation of continuing when you don't think you can.

- Resilience is digging deeper when you feel you have nothing left.

- Resilience is trying again regardless of how many times you failed before.

- Resilience is reframing each challenge as the beautiful opportunity it is.

- Resilience builds character. Character builds champions.

ASSIGNMENT: BUILDING RESILIENCE

Think about a time in your life when you worked hard for something and never gave up, despite plenty of obstacles and failures along the way. What things did you do every single day that ultimately led to you achieving your goal? Describe it in detail here:

>

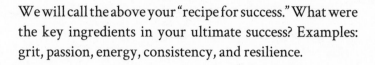

We will call the above your "recipe for success." What were the key ingredients in your ultimate success? Examples: grit, passion, energy, consistency, and resilience.

Think about a time when something didn't end up going the way you hoped it would.
Describe that time/event here:

What didn't you do in that situation that in hindsight you realize was necessary?

What aspects of your above "recipe for success" did you not use?

Think about something you are working hard to achieve right now. Describe it in detail:

What character traits or "ingredients" must you use in your "recipe for success" to achieve the above?

Are there tweaks to your original recipe that you will make for this one? What will those tweaks be?

What can you do today that helps build your resilience?

What must you stop doing?

What must you continue to do?

WHY does it matter to you?

Stay connected to that in every moment as that will be your FUEL!

Chapter 14

THE POWER OF HEALTH

One of the most important parts of the Power Line is Health.

Without our health we have nothing.

Hard to hear? Yes, it is. But I need to be very clear: without health, you have nothing.

All the things you love to do, the work that you do, and how you spend your time require health.

Do you want to be around for your child's wedding? Do you want to take those trips and have those adventures you have dreamed about with your friends? Do you want to continue doing the basic things you do every day? Well, then you MUST prioritize your health.

Leukemia brought me to my knees. Everything I loved to do, everything I dreamed of creating and bringing to life, I couldn't do. That was a reality hit that struck me hard and fast.

I remember as an athlete, if I got an injury, I would always ask myself, "What can I do?"

I didn't just stop all my training because I had a foot injury. So, I couldn't run. What else could I do?

I could swim more and more often. I could bike longer and harder. I could work on my mindset, my nutrition, and recovery.

If something takes you down, don't stop everything. Pivot and focus on the things you can do.

Leukemia was way more serious than a foot injury, knocking me down, but I would never let it knock me OUT.

Still in this situation, I asked myself, "What CAN I do?"

It became evident that this was giving me the opportunity to shed the parts of me that were no longer serving me.

My bone marrow transplant would not only wipe out the cancer within me, but it would remove it from my body forever.

The transplant would symbolize the removal of aspects in my mind, body, and spirit that needed to be let go of.

During this time, my focus was on releasing any guilt, resentments, anger, and anything negative that I had been harboring within. This challenge would force me to grow stronger with self-reliance. I reminded myself that I had the choice to accept or reject anything that I see, hear, or experience. Only I could decide to give it value and the power to affect my life.

The same is true for you.

I would take this time to master my mindset—my thoughts, my emotions, and the meaning I gave all that was happening to me.

I would discipline my focus in every moment by aiming high at what I wanted more than I have ever wanted anything before: my health and well-being.

Training to win this battle over leukemia was harder than any training I had ever done to become a world champion triathlete.

This battle for my health mattered more to me than anything ever had. It had to.

If I didn't win this battle, I wouldn't have all the things that mattered most to me in my life.

In LIFE there can be setbacks but NO RETREAT. When you persist, when you allow yourself to learn and grow from the setback, you then live life with no regrets.

I was going to see this sickness as a setback that, by facing it head-on and with belief in my ultimate triumph, would lead me to a better life. This would lead me to more of what I wanted: a deep connection with myself and with others and deeper love on every level.

This would be a time to rest, to go inside myself, and come back out when it was safe again.

During hard times, you need to take time and energy for yourself.

Withdraw into yourself and ask, "What do I need?"

Time for rest. Time to conserve your energy.

Time to reflect. Time to change something inside of you. Time to fill up with energy.

You will only know once you take this time for yourself.

I needed to heal. I needed to find an optimum balance of health between the mental, emotional, physical, and spiritual.

Being faced with my mortality, I would take this time where physically I was weak, sick, suffering, and under incomprehensible stress as an opportunity to heal my soul, connect deeply to my spirit, and strengthen my emotional and mental health.

Health is not just physical. It is emotional, mental, and spiritual.

What I realized through this experience is that when we take the time to prioritize all aspects of our health, the reward is beyond anything you can imagine.

Typically, physical health makes it easier to optimize your mental and emotional health. I didn't have that option. I would have to use my mental, emotional, and spiritual health to bring back my physical health.

You must step up to that challenge yourself.

Start with your mental and emotional health by taking ownership of the thoughts and focus you have.

Witness what certain thoughts make you feel. Witness the consequences of thinking that way. Then love yourself enough to redirect those thoughts so that they make you feel good, not bad; strong, not weak.

It is up to you.

Don't wait for a diagnosis to focus on your health.

Start now and the likelihood of you having to deal with a crisis becomes way less.

If you are faced with a crisis, your commitment to your health will provide you with the tools, strength, and belief to overcome it just as I did.

Do you want to feel better in any given moment? Rest your mind on things that make you feel good.

Love and appreciation: sink into these beautiful energies that are available to you all day.

Many times in my life I have used visualization to manifest the future I wanted.

As a young hack at triathlon, I would close my eyes and envision myself sailing through the water, effortlessly pounding the pedals of my bike, running like the wind, and being called a world champion at the finish line. I would literally see this happening as if it were real. I would FEEL all the feelings that would come along with that moment. I would hear what the people around me were saying.

Mom: "I am SO PROUD OF YOU!"

My coach: "YOU DID IT!"

My best friend: "I knew you had this in you!"

And me: "Wow, Siri. You did it. You are amazing. I love you."

I would use all my senses to create this manifestation in my mind and in doing so, I would feel the feelings that came along with it: joy, exultation, relief, and pride.

I felt that by doing this, my mind and soul would know exactly what we were working for every day.

This was something I "could do" every day while sick. Often what would inspire me to go there was hitting my emotional bottom, hitting my threshold for pain and sickness. This was my life preserver. I knew if I could take myself through this process, I would feel a little bit better.

I would close my eyes and I would picture myself running up my favorite mountain trail: the wind in my hair, the warmth of the sun on my cheeks, hearing my wife's voice behind me, laughing, feeling strong, feeling energized, getting to the top, and celebrating. I was fueled with vibrant health and energy. LIFE flowed through me. I experienced every single sensation I imagined. It was real to me, regardless of the fact that I was in a hospital bed fighting for my life.

A year and a half after my bone marrow transplant, I ran that mountain. It was just as I had experienced it in my mind thousands of times over the past two years.

I felt the wind on my face. Breathed in the crisp fresh mountain air. Laughed with my wife as we celebrated our great adventure. I got to the top, and I celebrated. I thanked God. Thanked all my angels and my guides, doctors, nurses, my umbilical cord donor, my sister, my mom, my wife, my dad, my chosen family, and MYSELF. I cried in gratitude. I was so beautifully full of the magnificent gift of life.

What you want most in life you must envision first in your mind.

If you need inspiration, start with vision boards.

It took me almost a full day to move into my hospital room. My mom and Bek were given the job of carrying all my posters and vision boards from the car to the eleventh floor, at which point they transitioned into decorators. I lay in my bed watching them, feeling so blessed to have their love and support.

I had every inch of my hospital walls covered in vision boards—pictures reminding me of what I was fighting for: runs up my favorite mountain trails with my wife, speaking events on Tony Robbins's stages, family vacations, horse riding, walks with my mom and along the beach with my Australian family, time with my best friend, training sessions with the athletes I coach, the horses Bek and I bring home after being rescued from the path to slaughter. These were pictures of me with my favorite people in the world. On the walls, there were also words of affirmation: BELIEVE. Gratitude. STRENGTH. Vibrant Health. Joy. Passion. Courage. Faith. Presence. LOVE.

These were all reminders of the life that awaited me—the life I would be living after conquering this beast.

This manifestation process is KEY to creating the future you dream of.

Get creative and don't hold back. Enjoy the feeling it gives you to be living the life that you've been dreaming of. This becomes the carrot that you move toward one step at a time, every day.

There is a gift in every struggle.

If you look back at your deepest struggles and search for the gift in them, you will undoubtedly find it.

I encourage you to do that often. In knowing this truth, you will carry that into any future challenge you face, and it will enable you to face it with more courage, faith, and grace.

Every single day I thought about the lessons in what I was going through. I had to find meaning in my pain and suffering. Doing so made me feel more in control of my fate.

If this was meant to teach me something, then I would figure out what that was so the lesson could be learned, and then I could be free.

That was my thought, and it served me well.

I will share with you the most profound gifts that revealed themselves through this terrifying, heart-wrenching, and agonizing challenge. These are gifts that I am forever grateful for, gifts so life-changing that I can honestly say, "I wouldn't change a thing about what has happened."

For all my life until now, I believed I needed to suffer to succeed.

That served me for a time but what I realize now is that I don't need to suffer any longer.

I am meant to live life effortlessly.

That doesn't mean there won't ever be painful times. Pain happens but suffering is a choice.

I choose NOT to suffer.

I choose to use the gifts of my mind, focus, heart, and intuition to navigate any future challenge with grace.

I choose to thrive effortlessly.

To truly heal, I had to allow myself to show my feelings and not let my superpower of staying strong and forging through things deny me the opportunity to feel my own sensitivity.

I am committed to being real with myself, letting my sensitivity show.

I allow myself to BE in every moment.

No one has a perfect mindset in every moment. My goal is to be the best that I can be in as many moments as possible and love myself through every moment.

It is so important that you be compassionate and loving with yourself.

Appreciate where you are at in every moment.

Love yourself through every moment—moments where your mindset is positive, present, grateful, appreciative, and totally focused on love and moments where you may be having a more difficult time. FLOW.

I learned the importance of self-love.

I loved myself through the tough moments and allowed my pain to be heard and acknowledged.

I realized the importance of knowing my innocence and releasing my guilt and self-judgment.

I learned just how important it was to receive and get my divine feminine energy flowing.

It is in receiving that we can GIVE SO MUCH MORE.

I became adept at having love and compassion for myself. I saw the beauty, love, light that is me.

I became aware of how loved I truly am, not just by others but by myself.

The power of love, gratitude, and compassion became so very clear.

I witnessed how my own consciousness, my infinite being, can heal.

I didn't need to suffer to achieve.

I didn't need to force things.

Life could be effortless if I lived from my heart.

It was important to refuse to buy into a negative belief system and know the truth.

I would hold love, gratitude, joy, healing, compassion, and all things high energy.

We have power over our own lives and knowing this reduces our overall anxiety and gives us a renewed sense of well-being and life.

I must live in love for love's sake: love for myself and for others.

All healing comes in a state of calm and joy. To get to this place, you must learn how to observe your inner state constantly. Be on the lookout for your inner critic and recognize its voice. Choose to lower the volume on that voice and increase the volume on your inner truth.

As you become aware of your inner critic, it loses its power over you.

This opens the door to you truly being able to orchestrate your feelings at any given moment. Choose to love over fear. Choose joy over despair. Choose gratitude over inadequacy.

It has been so important for me to become comfortable with all the parts of who I am—not just comfortable but to celebrate them. For I am unique. Just as you are. That is what makes us special.

When you remove judgment for yourself, you make room for joy, peace, and calm. These are emotions and feelings that put you in an optimal space for healing and thriving.

From this state, everything in life you can feel grateful for: the challenges and the good times. All of it is this beautiful gift of life.

It is in this state where maximum growth happens and your capacity for impact in the world magnifies.

This all starts with mindfulness. Take the time to be present with yourself. Listen to what you have to say: what you are feeling, what you need, what you must continue doing, what you must stop doing, and what you must start to do.

Then take that vision of what you want to experience in life and who you want to be and SEE THAT PERSON. SEE that LIFE. Feel what it feels like to be them. Feel what it feels like to be living that life.

This is all mindfulness.

So very powerful.

So where do you start with prioritizing your health?

It starts with appreciating your body for all it has done for you.

I used to really be hard on myself for my body. This was something I had to forgive myself for.

It all started during my triathlon career. At that point, I had a decent body image. I was so thankful for my body for getting out there every single day pushing itself to become faster, stronger, fitter, and better able to compete at the level I dreamed of. But then I went to Switzerland to train with Brett Sutton, the most decorated triathlon coach in the world.

He had coached multiple world champions and Olympic medalists. One of the first days I was at training camp, Brett had me step on a scale in front of the entire squad. As I stepped on the scale, he yelled out with a laugh, "Look at those rabbits in a sack."

I was horrified. He was talking about my thighs that had taken me from never having done a triathlon to competing as a professional six years later. I was horrified and hurt. I felt hurt for myself and for the amazing body that had done so much for me.

He proceeded to say that I would be on the lettuce team, which meant that I would follow his diet of just lettuce and salads, as I had at least ten to fifteen pounds to lose.

Ashamed and hurting, I was told to get in the pool. "Let Siri get in first. Otherwise, there might be a tidal wave if she gets in after you."

I did not find this funny.

I felt so alone. Cornered. Bullied. Ashamed.

I quickly jumped in the water so that people could no longer stare at my bottom and pass judgment on this body that I had loved and appreciated until that moment.

I cried in my goggles, contemplating whether this lettuce diet was really a thing.

Fortunately, I had a good head on my shoulders, and I would never take it so far to train six to eight hours a day and only give my body lettuce. I would not do that to myself. But I got the message. I needed to lose weight. I would tell him I was on the lettuce diet, but I would lose the weight in a way that felt healthy and kind to my body.

Every day was a constant tug of war between my love and appreciation for this amazing body of mine and this new truth that I was so deeply flawed, in my coach's opinion.

From that day forward, I never ever wanted anyone to look at me from straight behind.

Even in the first five years of my marriage to Bek, she had never seen my bottom straight on.

So sad. So very sad.

I found a balance that felt like I was honoring my body enough to let it know how grateful I was for the intense work it did for me every day. I would lie in my bath and run my hands over my feet, calves, thighs, shoulders, arms, and hands to thank every single part of my body for its strength, power, and resilience. This was my way of showing gratitude and love for this body that had served me so well.

As far as my diet went, I decided I would cut out all bread and starchy carbohydrates after breakfast. At breakfast, I would allow myself one piece of toast with either peanut butter or eggs. After that, I would only eat salads and lean proteins for every single meal.

These were big salads with all colors of the rainbow, low-fat cheese such as feta, cottage cheese, or goat cheese, and either chicken or fish with every meal.

Each week, I would get a thumbs up from Brett, saying, "that lettuce diet is working well!"

So proud of myself for losing the weight slowly but healthfully and with respect for my body.

Eventually, I got down to the weight he had recommended. He was right. I was lighter. I was stronger. I was faster. And I was ready to WIN.

Had I done it his way, I think physically, mentally, and emotionally I would be beat before even getting to the starting line. But the way I had managed it kept my health as the utmost important thing.

Fast forward to AML.

When you lose twenty-five pounds and don't have much energy to work out or build strength, your body changes dramatically. Loose skin, which suddenly seemed wrinkly, less muscle, and not a lot of shape. It was so far from the athletic, strong, muscular, and lean body that I had lived in for the past twenty-five years.

But this time, I didn't judge what my body looked like. That didn't matter anymore. Instead, I would look in the mirror and almost cry with gratitude for this incredible body that fought the most gruesome war from within. It withstood bombs dropped on it. It withstood a complete overhaul of my immune system. It had withstood AML, pneumonia, and severe gastric distress, which had often had me vomiting over sixty times in one day.

Yet here it was thriving. On the other side. This body may not be the muscles and tight skin that it used to be, but this body was the most awesome, beautiful, resilient, and strong body I could ever dream of having.

This body was a miracle and I will cherish for the rest of my life. I gave it the gratitude, exultation, and celebration that it so deserved.

What I went through was a gift, in that I let go of the judgment so wrongly placed on this incredible vessel of mine. I forgave myself for having felt the way I did about it back then as a professional athlete. I did the best that I could to take the information Brett gave me and not have that destroy my body image for life.

But here I am, so happy, so blessed to live in this body— this masterpiece.

What has your body done for you? Think about it. It has worked tirelessly to take you places you wanted to go. It has done all that you needed to get done to arrive right where you are now.

Start focusing on that. Be grateful. Celebrate the amazing body that has been your vessel for a lifetime and if you haven't already, start treating it with the love and respect it deserves.

Learn how to care for your body.

What will it take for you to achieve optimum health?

Must you start eating better like less processed foods, sugars, alcohol, and things that cause disease?

Must you drink more water and aim to alkalinize your blood through alkaline foods?

Must you start exercising to strengthen your heart, increase your energy, and elevate your mood?

Exercise alone is a game-changer.

The Sirius Squad, which is a fitness squad my wife and I developed, was formed to get people off the couch and onto their feet for a fifteen-minute workout every single day.

I had developed a bunch of plans that I was using with Melissa Etheridge. She was looking to get fit on tour but didn't have a lot of time to train. These fifteen-minute sessions were efficient, effective, fun, and addictive! They included multiple intervals going from a hard effort to an easy recovery, on any piece of equipment, or even just in your own home by using the stairs or walking in place.

Melissa got tremendous results with this training, so Bek and I decided to offer it to Etheridge Nation, the collective name of the hundreds of thousands of amazing humans who are Melissa's most loyal fans.

The Sirius Squad gained great momentum in changing people's lives. Some lost fifty to sixty pounds and loved the new healthy lifestyle that led to that.

Some got off pain meds after years of depending on them. Some got off blood pressure meds after years of needing them. Some got out of a wheelchair for the first time, strong enough to begin the road to walking again.

The results were mind-blowing, and Bek and I were so proud.

We saw people putting their health in their own hands. They made it a priority and then reaped the benefits of increased energy, which led to being more effective at work. This led to promotions or valuing themselves more and thus they moved on to work better suited to their higher energy and greater confidence.

These people were starting to love and appreciate themselves more. They were building confidence and their relationships were thriving because of this shift.

The physical benefit bled into the emotional and mental health of these people, and this was life-changing.

It all started with fifteen minutes a day.

The first step is to do these things:

1. Change the meaning you give exercise. It must be an empowering meaning so that you WANT to do it.
2. If you don't think you can do the whole session, just give me two minutes. Walk outside your door and give me two minutes. The key is to build up consistency. This consistency is what will allow you to build this into a habit, a lifestyle a love.
3. Celebrate after every session. We ask that everyone put a post on our Facebook page with a "BOOM!" signifying they did the workout and were celebrating their success. The community will respond with everyone celebrating each other's progress, creating an incredible energy of support and love.

Just start with one minute or two minutes. Just get out the door. Breathe in the fresh air and feel good about making a choice to put yourself first—your health first.

You are taking ACTION to improve your health. One minute is all it takes.

As you begin to feel the benefits of this commitment and the sense of well-being, confidence, and strength it brings, you will find yourself wanting to do more and more.

If you want specific guidance on this journey, you can join us at www.siriussquad.com.

Just like fitness compounding over time, so do bad habits.

You may think that you are healthy, energized, and doing great work, BUT you don't take good care of yourself as far as eating healthy or exercising.

Don't wait for a diagnosis to start taking care of your health.

Those bad habits are compounding over time, and although they haven't manifested in bad health, inevitably they will. Don't allow that to happen.

Take charge now. Build healthy habits little by little and the benefits from doing this will compound in a powerful way over time.

Treat your body like the luxury vehicle that it is, not like a rental car.

> "To give anything less than your best is to sacrifice the gift." — STEVE PREFONTAINE

You are the gift; your body is the gift. This life is the gift.

Decide to be the champion of your life in every single moment.

Love yourself, honor yourself, and care for yourself as you would your most beloved.

What you create from that space becomes your gift to the world.

Remember this:

- Don't treat your body like a rental car. Treat it like the luxury vehicle it is.

- Everything you want to do in your life requires health. Make health a priority!

- You GET to work out. You GET to eat healthy. You GET to prioritize health.

- Exercise will increase your energy, elevate your mood, increase your well-being, and build confidence and strength.

ASSIGNMENT: HEALTH

What do you want most in life?

Can you have that without health?

What does health mean to you?

What do you believe about health?

What have the consequences been in the past, having this belief?

What will the consequences of having this belief be in the future?

What must you stop doing?

What must you continue doing?

What must you start doing?

What must health mean to you to make it a priority?

What are some of your lifetime goals?

1.

2.

3.

Is your current state of health going to see you achieving those goals?

What must you believe about health to achieve those goals?

1.

2.

3.

What steps will you take TODAY to improve your health?

1.

2.

3.

What habits or rituals will you put in place in order make the above happen?

1.

2.

3.

What will be the rewards of taking this action? What gifts will this health bring into your life and the lives of those you love and care about?

Remember you are setting a beautiful example for your kids, friends, and family. You change your health for the better, they will witness how this changes your life, so they will want to do the same!

My wife and I offer a free seven-day challenge you can participate in to jumpstart your future health focus, NOW! Just visit our website siriussquad.com and get your fitness journey started today.

This is my gift to you.

It is important you take action right when you make the decision to make health a priority. That time is now.

Chapter 15

THE POWER OF FAITH

There is one thread that has run through the entire fabric of my life for as long as I can remember: FAITH.

This feeling that we are never alone. This feeling that somehow our lives are being guided by a power greater than us.

Faith, to me, is that invisible hand holding yours, moving beside you, and giving you the courage to take that next step.

Every August from when I was born until I was sixteen, my father would take my sister and me to Kennebunkport, Maine, one of the most beautiful places in the world. There was something so sacred about it. I would get a peaceful and soothing feeling when we drove past the sign: WELCOME TO KENNEBUNKPORT."

We would stay with my grandparents at their house on the river. I would sit for hours just watching the boats drive by, heading out for a wonderful adventure at sea. I would imagine the things they would see, the conversations they would have, and I would vicariously take joy in that experience.

Sitting out on our dock, I would hang my toes in the water and hope that fish would come by and kiss them. I would take in the warm embrace of the sun and the kisses of wind on my face.

My favorite time was Sunday morning when we would go to St. Ann's Episcopal Church for the early service at 6:00 a.m. and watch the sun rise over the ocean from the seaside chapel. It was an outdoor place of worship with an awe-inspiring view of the Gulf of Maine as a backdrop.

All I knew is that when I was in Maine, and especially at that church, I felt the arms of God and the angels around me.

I had never been to Bible study, never read the Bible, and had no real guidance on what that path would look like. As a kid, I felt too afraid to ask the question that I so desperately wanted the answer to. If this feels so good, why don't we do it more often? We went every Sunday in Maine but only went on Christmas and Easter at home.

Finally, at about age eleven, I said to my mom and dad, "I believe in something more. I want to get closer to that. Can we start going to church on Sundays?"

So, we did. I would go with my dad on the weekends I stayed with him and with my mom on the weekends with her. These are some of my most cherished memories with each parent.

I always wanted to go to the early service. The sun would be rising and as it did, the rays of light would pierce through the stained-glass windows. I would follow the lines of color as they rested on the people's faces and on my own. I found this so beautiful. God was shining his light on us.

I felt seen. I felt heard. I felt understood. In this place, I never felt alone.

As I began racing professionally in triathlon, my training took me away from those opportunities to show my thanks to this beautiful energy that gave me so much comfort. Most races happened on Sundays. I started using that day to truly be present while I was doing my long-run sessions, saying my prayers as I ran. I showed my gratitude by taking in the beauty of this amazing world we live in. "Wow, God. What you have created here is simply extraordinary. Thank you."

What I started realizing is that I found God in nature. I found God in animals: chirping birds, smiling dogs, resting cows in a pasture, and butterflies blessing our skies. Anytime I was out in nature, I would get the same feeling I got in church—that filling up, that peacefulness, that knowing that I am not alone.

There was a greater power at work that was not only creating this beautiful life that I lived, but it was also guiding me on this journey. It was setting me up to learn everything I needed to learn through experience. Everything I would carry into my future. It was equipping me to weather any storm and overcome any challenge. It was guiding me to all I needed to become to live the life I dreamed of.

I realized that this is FAITH.

It was a hand holding mine. It was a beautiful force not carrying me, but always walking beside me.

Faith was that extra set of hands that could help in times of need—that voice of encouragement when I felt tired or defeated.

Faith was the wind on my back that kept me going even when I didn't think I could continue.

With this faith, I found that I would take the risks necessary to reach all new levels in my sport. I would take risks that would give me the information I needed on whether to pursue a certain relationship or pathway in life.

Faith gave me the confidence to move forward despite my fear.

I could be afraid but do it anyway. Faith gave me courage.

That courage led me to prove to myself that when I did something, even if I didn't know that I could, it always led me to something great.

It was even something as simple as racing at the World Triathlon Championships in Edmonton, Canada. I dug deeper than I ever had before and experienced discomfort at a level totally foreign to me. But I was at the front of the race. This was my opportunity to find out what I was really made of. I was being pushed by the number one athlete at the time, Michellie Jones, who was running right on my shoulder, so I decided to go beyond anything I ever had done before. I clicked into another gear and took my level of effort from a ten to an eleven. Who knew there was an eleven?

Going to that place is what ultimately led me to become world champion that day. It took courage. It took faith in me—faith in my ability to withstand this level of suffering and follow it through to the finish line.

Faith is having complete trust or confidence in something without proof. It is conditioning and turning up the volume on that inner knowing that when you do all that is required to become the person you need to become, you will achieve that goal!

Faith begets faith. Faith in a greater power whether that be God, the universe, or Mother Nature, ultimately leads to you developing faith in yourself.

Faith is imperative on this journey as it goes beyond hope. Faith lives deep in your heart and spirit. In times of great struggle or sadness, faith is the KNOWING, deep down inside, that you are going to be okay, and this too shall pass.

The sun will rise again tomorrow.

Faith carried me through my battle with leukemia.

I wanted to document my journey on social media because I knew the power of love and the power of prayer could help me heal. I wanted people to know so if they so generously prayed for me, I would feel their prayers, and my progress would reflect them.

I was meant to be speaking at Tony Robbins's Date with Destiny event, my all-time favorite event of his. But, instead, I was headed to the hospital for my first treatment in the clinical trial. Tony and Sage sent me a box full of prayers and love notes from not only Robbins Research International, the company behind Tony and his amazing events, but also from all the participants. When I opened this box, I felt the love pouring out of it. I felt the strength and power in those prayers.

My mom, every single night, would kneel by my bed, take my hands, and pray. Tears rolling down my eyes, I would melt into those moments with my mom, feeling her heart pouring into her prayers for me. I was so deeply touched and so comforted by her devotion and love.

I will never forget my dear friend Sage Robbins calling me in the hospital. She asked me how I was, and I replied honestly that I didn't know if I had what it took to see this through. I was disillusioned by everything I was going through and terrified and folding under the sheer exhaustion of navigating this road.

I was so tired I couldn't even pray. She said, "Siri, in times like these, the only prayer you have to say that God will hear is 'God, please help me.'"

So, I did, and God heard my prayers. I felt the presence of light and love around me. I felt a greater strength just knowing that I didn't have to do it all on my own.

Sage was such a beacon of light for me during this time and continues to be.

The prayerfulness we shared connected us in the most profound way.

I would call her for prayers before any major procedure. She would guide me with the most beautiful words of grace and comfort. I truly felt as though the Lord was speaking through her. She gave me this extraordinary gift that fortified me in every way.

Before every treatment, I would read the prayers Sage had sent me. The nursing staff and doctors would often sit in for the prayer. These moments left me feeling so guided and supported, and they strengthened my faith to a level I had never experienced before.

At every treatment was this prayer:

> Oh, Heavenly Father, thank you for
> the miracle of healing my body.
>
> Thank you for this medicine
> being a blessing, Lord.
>
> I just thank you for guiding us
> and perfecting my cells.

Thank you for filling my body with light now.

Oh, Heavenly Father, every doctor, every nurse,
that comes in, please bless them, God. If they are
in front of me, they are angels and are a gift.

Oh, Heavenly Father, I thank you
for holding me in the light.

I thank you for surrounding me.

I thank you for renewing my body,

Renewing my cells.

I thank you for the resurrection of every
cell in my body and entire system.

Oh, Heavenly Father, thank you for this
medicine being such a blessing to my system
and the miracles continuing to unfold.

I thank you, Lord, for blessing me and guiding the
doctors, physicians, and nurses, and my family.

Thank you for surrounding me
with such light, Lord.

We trust in you.

We give all our burdens and
worries and fears to you.

Lord, just at the altar of our faith,

Each breath we take we just breathe in more
light and release what is no longer needed, Lord.

Thank you for filling me with
such beautiful light.

Thank you for being with us.

Thank you for holding us,

Surrounding us,

Amen 🙏💜

I will be forever grateful for Sage's love and guidance. She is truly an angel on this earth.

Tony Robbins has lit the path for me since I was twenty years old. He guided me through his works including books, cassette tapes, interviews, and simply through his example in this world. He is the most loving, kind, generous, and wise man I have ever known. I owe him a debt of gratitude. Every word I read, I put into action in my own life. It became my *modus operandi*. His works became my personal manifesto. Tony has been my guide for the last thirty years. His work in this world is transformative. He single-handedly is making this world a better place. I am me because he is. I really believe that. Sage, his incredible wife, has brought me spiritual guidance that I leaned on heavily throughout my AML journey and carry forth into every moment of this miracle of life now.

Mary Buckheit, another incredible member of this family, instilled in me the faith that your chosen family will always live in your heart in every single moment. I can infinitely draw from that space the love, strength, and guidance that nourishes my soul and fills me with joy. Right after being diagnosed, Mary brought me a box of books that she had read that she knew would help fill me with hope, insights, strength, and faith. With every page I read, I felt Mary with me. Highlighted sentences seemed to be exactly what I needed to hear in that moment. It was as if she was there with me, pointing out all the things that would help me heal. She was keeping me focused on my dream of SURVIVAL.

In the toughest times of my illness, I often had this deep sensation of a presence along with me. Always. I was never alone. This I know was my idea of God.

God doesn't have to mean the same to you as He/She means to the people around you.

YOU get to go FIRST in deciding what this higher power is—what it means to you and how you appreciate it.

You get to GO FIRST in deciding to let this energy in or to pretend it's not there.

My advice to you is to let it in. This light source, this energy source, is all LOVE.

Acknowledge the gift. Embrace the gift. Live with that gift in your heart in every moment.

If you choose to believe, you too can be awed by the gift of these messages.

Faith fills my heart and soothes my soul. Faith is the hand I will hold every moment for the rest of my life.

In the Power of Health chapter, I spoke about visualizing or manifesting the outcome you want to reach: the future you that you want to be.

Faith is having a strong belief in the vision you create in your mind, of yourself already having accomplished your goal. Put yourself in that moment as if it were happening NOW. What are you doing? Who is with you? What are you saying? What are they saying? How do you feel? Play out the celebration in your mind.

This all requires FAITH: faith in yourself and faith in your ability to do what might seem impossible. It is having trust and confidence in something without being offered any proof.

Without faith, you may not even entertain the possibility.

Without faith, it may be too scary to even try.

Develop this faith in your life and you will see how remarkably it strengthens you from the core, the hope it brings, the courage it inspires, and the miracles it manifests.

My eyes are always open to the signs I receive from the universe, and from God and my angels.

My beloved soulmate dog Calvin passed away four years ago and, to this day, I miss him so much. From the day he died, he would send me messages. My phone would be off in the middle of the night as I slept and suddenly music would start playing loudly, waking my wife and me up. Bek would say, "Why in the world did you do that?!" I explained it wasn't me. The songs that played were not even in my library, but the words meant so much. It was obvious that this was his way of letting me know he was with me always.

I even started a playlist called "Calvin's Playlist" which includes all the songs that would play out of the blue, whether sleeping or going about my day.

Here is the playlist:

"Couldn't Ask for a Better Friend" by Michael Logen

"Love Is Bigger Than Anything in Its Way" by U2
"Angel" by Aerosmith
"Run To Me" by Bee Gees
"Bridge Over Troubled Water" by Simon & Garfunkel
"Float On" by Modest Mouse
"If" by Bread
"Seven Bridges Road" by Eagles
"Leader of the Band" by Dan Fogelberg
"Leather and Lace" by Stevie Nicks & Don Henley
"Don't Cry" by Guns N' Roses
"All Summer Long" by Kid Rock
"Our House" by Crosby, Stills, Nash, & Young

As you can see, Calvin has incredible taste in music.

Now, whenever I see a butterfly around my head while walking or running, I say, "Hi, Calvin! I love you SO MUCH!"

Or when I walk right over a feather, I know it is him.

Whomever you think of in that moment when you are getting your sign is who is there with you. This is what I believe.

This is what I KNOW.

Open your eyes to the signs you receive daily: signs of support, signs that a loved one who has passed is watching over you, signs that you are on the right track, and signs that you are not.

Give yourself permission to enjoy the conversation that happens as the universe supports you in finding your way to all that you dream of in life.

Remember this:

- In times of great struggle or sadness, faith is the KNOWING, deep down inside, that you are going to be okay and this too shall pass.

- Give yourself permission to enjoy the conversation that happens as the universe supports you in finding your way to all that you dream of in life.

- Faith in a greater power builds faith in yourself.

- Faith is that invisible hand holding yours, moving beside you, and giving you the courage to take that next step.

ASSIGNMENT: EXPLORING YOUR FAITH

Have you ever felt guided in your life? Describe the times when you felt guided.

Do you believe in signs? What signs have you received in your lifetime that helped you plan your next steps? Or signs that signified you were not alone?

Please describe in detail.

Do you believe in some higher power or greater source of energy in your life? How would you describe it?

What does it mean to you?

How can you make your relationship stronger with that energy?

How will that benefit your life?

What does FAITH mean to you?

What must happen to have faith in yourself?

What is in your life now that you only dreamed of before?

Describe in detail and take a moment to really feel the gratitude, the appreciation, the pride, and the celebration in this reality.

Never take for granted the amazing work you have done in your life—the magic you have created. Celebrate and appreciate these things.

This will allow you to create even more with faith, belief, confidence, and courage.

Top 3:

    1.

    2.

    3.

What other things can you appreciate about the progress you have made or what you have created in these different aspects of your life?

    1.

    2.

    3.

List 3 major challenges you have overcome.

    1.

    2.

    3.

The above is your proof! It is proof of the things you have created in your life, the challenges you have overcome, the things you have achieved.

By stacking your proof, I hope you find that you have every right to have faith in YOU: your abilities, your decisions, and your actions.

Chapter 16

THE POWER OF LOVE

I saved the most important Power Line for last. If you are going to free yourself to truly create the masterpiece of life you desire, you must LOVE.

Love is the most beautiful source of energy that will carry you through the darkest of times.

It is in loving yourself that you want more for yourself.

It is in loving yourself that you will lean into difficulty, knowing the reward on the other side.

It is in loving others that we are, in turn, loved. This love inspires. This love emboldens. This love transforms.

Love truly does heal.

When my extraordinary wife came into my life, it changed me forever.

I finally had found a love for myself and was ready to love her in all the ways she so deserved—unconditionally, with vulnerability, and with every ounce of my soul wanting to light her up.

The most beautiful way to express love is with no expectation of getting anything in return. Just loving for the sake of loving. Love because of how good it makes the other person feel and how good that makes you feel.

At the time, I wasn't looking for someone to "complete" me. I had finally realized that I was complete all on my own. I was whole. I didn't need another person to make me that way.

Once you understand that, you can then step into the adventure of love without an expectation of getting something and instead, your only concern becomes what you can give.

This perspective alone is the seed that brings life to an extraordinary relationship.

When you have two people who just want to light up the other person's life, you end up getting all that you ever wanted and needed without even asking for it.

When we love deeply, it is natural for the receiver of our love to want you to feel the same. The act of love is what fills us up, and in filling up, we yearn to fill up another.

My wife quickly became my muse. Every single day she inspired me to want to be the very best version of myself for her, for the world, and for myself.

Her support and unbridled love have given me confidence and energy that I had never felt before.

The past several relationships, most of which left me feeling beaten and exhausted, convinced me that I would never ever be enough for another person.

Right before staying together in Australia with Bek, who at the time was my athlete, I had made a vow to myself that I would never again enter a relationship that wasn't EVERYTHING I had ever dreamed it to be: one of unconditional love and mutual respect. It would be one where we would lift each other up, encourage each other to shine our lights brighter than ever before, become more together, share great adventures, and love with no limits.

At the time, I had resigned myself to the belief that the relationship that had checked off all those things was with my dogs. I was okay with that.

A month later, I see this woman I had known for fifteen years in a totally different light. I got to know Bek the human, not just the athlete. As the months went by, it became clear. I didn't want to live another day without this woman in my life, by my side, and in my heart. She was the other pea in my pod. She was the wind beneath my wings, and I the wind beneath hers.

Our love for one another has healed the wounds of our past and strengthened our capacity to love others. Our love for one another has manifested into an energy that has led to us being unstoppable as a couple. We are unstoppable in our mission to make this world a kinder, more loving, and more compassionate place.

She is the most beautiful gift I have ever received.

It's an unexpected gift—but one that I will cherish for a lifetime.

Her love is one of the things that gave me the will to live, to survive AML.

My love is for her, my family, and our horses.

Love gives us purpose. Love gives us strength that is undeniable.

Please don't ever say no to love.

Even if it is temporary, it is always well worth the time spent.

It is in love that we strip ourselves down to the rawest and most vulnerable versions of who we are. It is like a tree shedding all its leaves in the fall. That shedding, becoming naked and vulnerable, leads us to a beautiful blossoming—a becoming. We can become a truer version of ourselves, connecting at the deepest levels to who you are. What you desire, what you dream of, what fears lie deep within, and what must be done to dance with those fears—move forward with these thoughts and open yourself up to the rich possibilities that lie ahead when you do so.

Love draws out the magic in the person to whom it is directed.

I have seen this with the horses we rescue. I have seen it throughout my life with people. When you express your love to another, they are reminded of the best parts of themselves.

When I decided to live my life from a place of love and not fear, it changed EVERYTHING for me.

Choose to LOVE every aspect of life—the good times, the bad times, the victories, and the failures—because life is a miracle. We are ALIVE. It feels so much better to love than to hate. Embrace the challenges and find the good in them rather than meet them with resistance, anger, and frustration.

When you approach the world around you with love, it changes your perspective. It changes how you see things. From a lens of love, you can truly witness the magic that is all around us. You are more apt to see the good, rather than the bad. You are more likely to feel happy, not sad.

Every single day, I witness the love my mom puts out into the world. It awes me. She owns and runs The Pampered Pooch in Boulder, Colorado. The care and love she shows every person and dog that enters is so inspiring. You can see the shift in the energy that my mom's presence brings immediately. The dogs want to stay, and the people always want to come back.

She embodies acceptance, patience, tolerance, and unconditional love.

She will take hours with a nervous dog. One snip of hair, stop, snuggle, love on them, and repeat.

The next time the dog comes in for grooming, they literally RUN to the door to come in.

My mom wants every human being to feel accepted and to know love, her love.

My mom reminds me every day how loved I am and how my presence in this life matters. She says how she feels. She expresses her love, and it is the most beautiful gift I could ever ask for.

My wife's mom Ruth does the same. She always comes from a place of love. From the first day we met, Ruth welcomed me into her family with open arms. She saw me. She accepted me. She believed in me. This gave me the courage to fight for this love that had struck me like no other. Her love was the permission I needed to believe in my ability to love her daughter as I dreamed.

Bek and I are both so blessed to have these beautiful examples of unconditional love. So much of who our moms are and how they make us feel is why we both are the way we are today.

When I told my mom I was gay, she responded with a hug saying, "I love you no matter what you are, because all you are to me is you."

Every single day she finds a way to guide me to know my value, my worth, my beauty, and my magic. Every single day.

I find myself doing the same.

Love breeds more love. Give without holding back and open yourself to receiving in the same way.

If you love someone, tell them. If you have something nice to say, say it.

Don't hold back your love. It is the elixir of life.

Tony and Sage Robbins have always said, "Relationships are a place you go to give, not to get."

This is so very true.

It is in loving that we feel loved, and it is in loving so generously, without expectation of getting anything in return, that love is brought back to us in kind.

I believe you MUST love others, and even harder, you MUST love yourself. If you're going to back yourself and choose to live your dreams, you must believe that you are worthy of that kind of goodness. And that comes from love.

This was a hard lesson for me. With every experience, it became more and more clear that the love I had been craving for a lifetime was my own.

It couldn't come from my parents, another human, or my animals. What I craved most was to feel that love from me to myself.

I asked myself constantly throughout the day, "What can I appreciate about myself in this moment? Or how can I love myself in this moment?"

Amid an argument, a moment of fear, or feeling overwhelmed, I ask myself, "How can I love myself in this moment?"

It became my guide to better support myself through the tougher moments in everyday life.

Once I gave myself permission to feel and express love for myself, I truly began to live, and my capacity to love grew in astounding ways.

I felt myself feeling love for a perfect stranger, an old lady who got all dressed up to do her grocery shopping. I adored how beautiful she looked and the pride she took in herself. This would almost make me cry with LOVE for her. I allowed myself to start feeling emotions like this.

I loved seeing one of our Sirius Squad athletes, who had never worked out in their life, taking on one of our fifteen-minute sessions. They faced their fears and dug deeper than they could ever imagine. They cried tears of pride after finishing successfully. In that moment, I felt such love for that person.

My desire to live with love led me to always look for what I loved about people, our world, and this life.

For example, if you believe that life is hard, then you will always find things that prove that life is hard. You will look for the challenge in everything and anticipate bad things happening. All of this proves your belief right.

Change the meaning of "life" to "LIFE IS A GIFT." You will always be present to all the gifts of this beautiful life with each breath: the opportunities for growth, the moments of celebration, the tenderness of relationships, and the wonder of nature. The meaning you give life then leads you to focus on all the proof that this belief is true.

Imagine the power of changing "love is cruel" to "love is kind." How would this change the way you love?

When I made the decision to love myself, I had to rewrite my "old story" from "It is so hard for me to love myself" to "There is so much to love about me. I love myself with all my heart."

Did I believe that in that moment? No, I didn't, but I was willing to lean into the discomfort of role-playing this new story until I became that version of me that truly loved herself.

I had to build habits and rituals into my daily life to support this new story, like waking up in the morning, putting my hand on my heart, and asking myself, "What do I love and appreciate about myself?" I made sure that I didn't give the same answers every day, and instead, got creative in truly exploring the things I appreciated about myself.

I then went into the bathroom and looked at myself in the mirror, right into my eyes. I held my gaze and from my heart said, "I love you, Siri."

This may seem silly, but it is necessary. You must develop new habits and rituals to support this love for yourself.

So many of us have been caught in patterns of self-judgment, self-deprecation, and mistreatment of the most important person: ourselves.

The more you tell yourself how imperfect you are, how broken you are, how unskilled you are, how unlovable you are...the more you begin to believe it. You are hammering this into your mind, and you hear it so often that it becomes what you think is your truth.

It is NOT. It is time to wake up to the truth: your imperfections are what make you unique. Embrace them and you will find that they are your superpower.

You are not broken; you are whole and always have been.

You are having a human experience like everyone else in the world. You are handling it with strength, courage, and bravery and will develop even more magic within you because of it.

You may be unskilled in some areas but as you have proven, you have an enormous capacity to become great at whatever you choose to put your heart and soul into.

We can't expect to be skilled in something we don't work at mastering. But, if you want to get good at something that inspires you, love yourself enough to start from square one and learn what you must learn. Practice what you need to practice to become proficient and successful at that thing you want to do.

You are so loveable. Think of how deeply you have loved in your life. Think of the people, experiences, and animals you have loved, and all the love you have generously shared from your beautiful heart.

Look down at your two hands. Really study them. As you do, think about all that these hands have done throughout your lifetime. Who have they held? Who have they helped? What have they created and what work have they done? Feel the love and appreciation that comes from just sitting with that for a few moments.

What does it take for you to love and care about another person?

Do they have to achieve something extraordinary?

Do they have to have a certain amount of money in their bank account?

Do they have to have thousands of social media followers?

Do they have to be perfect?

Do they have to have the perfect body, face, hair, and clothes?

I know you will answer NO to all those questions.

So, why are the rules different for you to be loved?

Why do you think that you should have all the above to be loveable?

YOU DON'T!

So, think about the people you love most in your life. What do you love about them?

Now, look at yourself. Are you all those things too?

This is your PROOF that you deserve your own love as much they deserve it.

It is time to start recognizing all the reasons why you must acknowledge and appreciate your love for yourself.

Finally express that love to yourself.

Finally speak to yourself, treat yourself, and believe in yourself like you would your most beloved.

It is never too late. Start NOW.

One person in my own life who I want this for more than anything is my beautiful sister Lisa.

Lisa is the most loving human being I have ever met. She loves people and animals so deeply. She lives to make others happy. She lives to fill others with love. Remember, she saved my life. She gave me life.

But she doesn't do the same for herself. The love she shows others she has never allowed to give back to herself. Because of this, she has fallen into habits that are slowly killing her.

At eighty-four pounds and hanging on for dear life, I know the only thing that will save her. She has to decide to be the hero of her own life. She has to decide to love herself enough to fight to live, to believe in a future of purpose and joy, and to believe in herself.

I love my sister with all my soul. I want her to FIND A WAY through this life-threatening situation she is in. I pray that she, like you, can look in the mirror into her own eyes and see the beautiful human being that she is. I want her to see the little girl that has been craving her own love for a lifetime and finally open her arms to embrace her, love her, and be her own hero.

I love you, Lisa, and I believe in you.

There is an amazing book written by Gary Chapman. It is a brilliant book that has saved marriages and improved relationships all over the world.

According to Gary, there are five ways that people express their love for each other:

1. Gift giving
2. Words of affirmation
3. Physical touch
4. Quality time
5. Acts of service

In the beginning of any relationship, most people show their love in all five languages. This feels amazing, thus the term "honeymoon period." You just feel so deeply IN LOVE and are showing it and receiving it in every form. As the relationship grows, each person typically defaults to their primary love language.

This often leads to one partner saying, "You don't show me that you love me," while the other partner says, "I show you my love every single day."

This happened with my wife and me early on in our relationship.

Bek's most fluent love language is acts of service. Mine is words of affirmation.

So, I would show my love for her in the way I always felt loved. I would write love notes every morning that I would place next to her coffee cup. I would tell her a hundred times a day how much I loved her.

She would clean the house, make our bed, do the dishes, and clean the counters. She would pick up the hay for the horses, clean the barn, and clean up after the dogs.

We had a conversation one night when I said I just don't feel like you love me like you used to. She felt the same.

You see, in the beginning, we did ALL the things for each other and with each other. But, as time went on, we defaulted back to our primary love languages without talking about it, and we both were feeling less loved.

We discussed our love languages and realized that for Bek to feel loved, I needed to start loving in her language, so that meant more acts of service. For me to feel loved, I needed her to offer me more words of affirmation.

She started leaving me love notes by my tea and I started vacuuming, doing the laundry, sweeping the barn, filling her car up with gas, and taking it to the car wash.

Suddenly, our LOVE was alive again!

The thing is, though, it never died.

We just weren't loving each other in the language we each understood.

The shift this awareness can have in your relationships is profound.

I took this book to the next level by applying it to myself.

How can I best show my love for myself?

Words of affirmation: I looked into my eyes in the mirror and told myself how much I loved myself and how proud I was of who I am.

Quality time: I did things I loved to do every day. These were activities that brought me joy and filled me up, like taking my dogs for a walk, doing my gratitude ritual out by the lake, riding my horse, or just lying in the grass and being present with the beauty of this planet. I decided to schedule quality time with myself every single day.

I didn't just want to love myself better, I wanted to experience that honeymoon period that we do in relationships with others. So, I expressed my love for myself daily in more ways than one.

For physical touch, every night, I wrapped my arms around myself. I hugged myself and said thank you for the effort I put into the day, the work I did, how deeply I loved, and the joy I brought into the world around me. Or I thanked myself for being so brave and for staying strong amid a very tough, emotional day.

If during the day I ever felt insecure, scared, or in need of support, I took my own hands together and held them. I felt the love and support that it gave me—from me to me.

These are all habits that you, too, can put into motion to get comfortable with expressing that entirely deserved love for yourself.

At the end of this chapter, I have attached the five love languages assignment that will help you incorporate this into your relationships with family members, your spouse, your friends, or with YOURSELF!

We often spend our lives "looking for love."

It's like having your glasses on your head, you're looking EVERYWHERE for them, and you just can't find them. Suddenly, you realize, they have been on your head all along.

Love has been INSIDE OF YOU all along.

It has always been there. You have been looking for it everywhere else but right there IN you.

When we love, we are loved.

That love we feel for another comes from within us.

It is who we are.

It is why we are here.

Our ability to love others begins with our willingness and ability to love ourselves.

For we can only love others as much as we love ourselves.

When we can unconditionally accept ourselves for who we are and embrace our authenticity, then we can become free to truly tap into the endless supply of love we hold within.

Love without judgment.

Love without expectation.

Love with total acceptance for this beautiful masterpiece that is YOU!

When we can accept and love ourselves without judgment, we then bring that same quality of love to our relationships. It is the beautiful release of all the ties, holds, and anchors that keep us from loving with no bounds.

You say, "That is impossible. At least for me."

But is it? Is that true? Do you have proof that that is the case? That you simply cannot love and accept yourself?

NO, that is a decision you have made. A belief you have. A story you tell.

You get to go first in deciding how you want to live this life.

Do you want to live life hammering yourself and beating yourself up over not being perfect when no one on the planet is?

Or...

Do you want to fully embrace all the beauty, magic, and uniqueness that makes you, you?

Set yourself free to truly live life on your terms and create the masterpiece of life you so deserve.

The decision is in your hands.

You can make that decision NOW.

I WILL LOVE MYSELF UNCONDITIONALLY for the rest of my life.

I have a process that I have shared with my clients, and it is so incredibly powerful.

If you are ready to finally stop judging yourself, comparing yourself, doubting yourself, and resenting yourself, it is time to COMMIT TO YOU.

It is a lifelong commitment, like saying yes to marrying your soulmate. This commitment carries that same weight. That same importance. That same sanctity.

It is time to write your vows to you. Turn it into a ceremony.

Make it a memory that will last for a lifetime.

Buy yourself a ring. Frame your vows. Make it real.

Here is an example from one of my amazing clients, Laila, who did this process. She claims this has changed her relationship with herself and her life and she wanted to share it with you:

- When I see you smile, I can face the world.
- Because of your love, I feel like I can do anything and for that, I promise myself to you.
- I promise to live in truth with you and to communicate fully and fearlessly.
- I promise to seek a deep understanding of your wishes, your desires, your fears, and your dreams.
- I promise to nurture those dreams because through them, your soul shines.
- I promise to encourage your compassion because that is what makes you unique and wonderful.
- I promise to live fearlessly authentic, especially when it isn't easy.
- I promise to make you laugh when you are taking yourself too seriously.
- I promise to savor every moment, even the smallest ones.
- I promise to keep our life exciting, adventurous, and full of passion.
- I promise to stand by you, challenge you, and make each tomorrow the best it can be.

- From this day forward, you will never walk alone.
- I believe in you and no matter what happens out there, I've got your back.
- I love you so much—always.

Here are the vows another amazing client of mine, Lisa, wrote for herself:

- I will love you, hold you, and honor myself.
- I promise to encourage your compassion because that is what makes me unique and wonderful.
- I promise to nurture my dreams because my soul shines with dreams.
- I promise to be loyal and to put myself before others.
- I promise to laugh more when I take things too seriously.
- I will love you every minute of the day.
- I will be proud of everything I have done in my life because I have done more than so many people.
- I will let Lisa be Lisa and be proud of that.
- I know I will go through peaks and valleys, but I will still survive and come back stronger.
- My body is my temple, and I will not judge myself on my size because I am so strong.
- I will stop and enjoy all the beautiful things that I have in my life and not compare myself to others.
- I will cherish the little things and not just let them slip away.
- The present is today, the past is gone, and tomorrow is a gift—it's time to live today.
- I will learn to forgive so that I can live a true and happy life.

- The small things are small things, and I won't make them into mountains.
- I will start to be more open with the people whom I love and start to chip away some of the walls that I have built.

With these vows to myself, today is a new day filled with love, dreams, joy, and excitement. ♥ ♥ ♥ ♥ ♥

And finally, Ciska's vows:

Dearest Ciska,

- I will never stand between you and your dreams.

- I will always treat you with loving kindness and celebrate the divine being you are.

- I will never use negative or derogatory words when having conversations with you.

- I will always be on your side and have your back.

- I love and accept you completely and unconditionally for this life and for eternity.

- You are a star. ⭐

> With love and devotion,
> Ciska

I got married to myself on 16 October 2021 on the beach in Provincetown, Massachusetts. I placed beach pebbles on top of one another as a symbol of my vows, and I gave myself a ring. I then went on a five-day rim-to-rim hike in the Grand Canyon for my honeymoon. At the bottom of the canyon, on Bright Angel Trail, I swam under the sacred Ribbon Falls as a symbol of cleansing rebirth. —Ciska

Now, it's your turn.

Remember this:

- LOVE HEALS ALL.
- Live life from a place of LOVE, not fear.
- Love yourself in the language that you understand.
- Love others in their language.
- Relationships are a place you go to give, not a place you go to get.
- LOVE has been inside of you all along.

ASSIGNMENT: THE FIVE LOVE LANGUAGES WORKSHEET

Part One

List at least five things that you think make your part-ner, a friend, or a family member feel loved. Remember that it doesn't matter whether you understand why this makes them feel loved. The only thing that matters is the way that it makes them feel.

Your partner's/or significant person in your life's things that make them feel loved:

1.

2.

3.

4.

5.

Now list five things that make you feel loved. Do not question these things of yourself nor feel any guilt about them. You know how important these things are to you. Look at your first list and try to understand that the other person feels the same way about their own things. It does not matter why each of you feels this way. Your lists will most likely be different and this represents the different love languages.

Your own things:

1.

2.

3.

4.

5.

Part Two

Each day, for the next five days, do at least one of the things on the list for your loved one to make them feel loved. Do so selflessly with only the goal of making them feel loved, regardless of how awkward or uncomfortable it may make you feel. Keep a journal of how they reacted and of how it made you feel. **Fill in your journal entries here.**

After five days, talk with your loved one and tell them the five things that make you feel loved.

They, like most people, assume that what makes them feel loved also makes others feel loved. If you give them the opportunity to make you feel loved in your own way, then your relationship will grow to new levels.

Enter details of how this discussion went. How did you feel? And how did your partner react?

Part Three

Love yourself every single day in your primary love language.

What will you do?

EXTRA CREDIT: Writing your Vows

It is time to commit to YOU!

Your lifelong relationship with yourself will be the most powerful, important, and incredible relationship you will ever have.

It is time to write vows to yourself. Cherish and care for this relationship with yourself as you would your relationship with your most beloved.

What commitments will you make?

How will you treat yourself? Love yourself? Speak to yourself? Support yourself?

What do you promise to do for yourself during times of struggle or tough times?

What will you NOT do? Be creative.

Take your time to really think about what you want to feel and experience the rest of your life with YOU.

How do you need to show up to create that?

This may require a few rough drafts. Take your time and really try to create a masterpiece here. You deserve that!

Once you have written your vows, it is time to have a ceremony.

You can do this in front of the mirror or outside in a beautiful place. Read the vows to yourself with presence, feeling, emotion, and love. Symbolize this commitment with a ring or piece of jewelry. It should be something that can symbolize this incredible bond you are committing to today.

Chapter 17

PAYING IT FORWARD

After twenty years of coaching triathlon, I started feeling as though I had achieved all I had wanted to do in that arena. I started life coaching four years ago and found it exhilarating in every way.

This type of coaching had me on my toes constantly. I was facing different challenges with different people and really needed to grow at light speed to be who I needed to be to help my clients achieve the goals they came to me with.

Coaching triathletes had never been just about coaching swimming, biking, and running. I had always coached my athletes holistically, focusing on mind, body, and spirit.

But mindset stuff seemed to always be the athlete's minor, not major, focus in the process.

I always wanted to focus on the emotional, mental, and spiritual journey, and sometimes this caused concern for my athletes that didn't want me to stray from what they felt most important: the swimming, biking, and running.

But you see, for me, it's not about that. For me, it is about WHO YOU BECOME along the journey of becoming a triathlete.

For me, triathlon was the vehicle through which I found myself, found a belief in myself, found trust in myself, and found worthiness from within.

Triathlon was the breeding ground for the tools and strategies I would develop that would ultimately help me navigate through everything that would come my way in the future, beyond the sport.

In the spring of 2022, one of the top athletes in triathlon reached out, wanting to spend some time with the horses. She had heard about the incredible healing power of these beautiful beings and found herself in desperate need of help.

I, of course, was happy to oblige. Seeing how these horses have healed hundreds of people on our ranch alone, I knew they could give her the support she needed.

It turned out she had fallen into a deep depression. She was overcome with anxiety and suffered deeply with her mental health. Everywhere she went, she was told that she had severe depression, anxiety, and bipolarism and needed to go somewhere to get treatment for her myriad of problems.

After having spent a few hours with her at the ranch, I just saw this amazing athlete exhausted from ten years of training with no breaks. She was coming down from the high of a supreme performance at the World Triathlon Championship and realizing that the OUTCOME doesn't change you. Ever.

We think that achieving a certain goal will somehow change us, how we feel, or change our lives in some magical way.

It doesn't. You wake up the next day the same person you were the day before.

If you didn't have a greater purpose behind achieving that goal, you will find yourself having succeeded but not feeling

fulfilled. It's a horrible letdown after the dedication and sacrifice you put into the goal.

As Tony Robbins says, "Success without fulfillment is the
ultimate failure," and it feels that way. Although most can't put
into words this emptiness they feel once the goal is achieved.

I remembered feeling just as this athlete did many times in
my career. I knew that what she was experiencing was not a
severe mental disorder but a temporary depression that came
with the anticlimactic feelings after a major victory.

She was exhausted. She was burned-out and had fallen
prey to social media's pressure to be perfect. Social media
makes success look so easy—you just need the perfect form,
musculature, and training program.

So you, the viewer, are struggling every step of the way,
working your ass off, digging deeper than you could imagine.
It doesn't look easy for you. It feels anything BUT easy, and
you start to wonder, "What's wrong with me?"

You realize you are far from perfect. You are somehow
blinded from the truth that NO ONE IS PERFECT.

Without embracing the truth, you are left feeling worthless, less than, and under extreme pressure to somehow become
this perfect version of whatever it is you dream of being.

This is impossible. No one is perfect.

Yet somehow these images tap into our deepest wounds,
our greatest fears, and LOCKS in. They prove to us that we
were right, we don't matter. We are not enough, and we won't
be loved as we are.

This incredible human and athlete came to me living the
story that she had lost her mind. She was totally depressed,
overcome with anxiety, and there was no way out except

to check in to a place that could deal with all these problems she had.

It was destroying her relationships, her well-being, and her life.

She had been focusing on everything she didn't have, everything that was wrong, and all her perceived problems. She was focusing on everything over which she had no control: other people, what they do, what they think, how they respond, and how they react.

She was listening to what everyone else was telling her about her. You are sick. You need help. You are bipolar. You need lithium. There was a big lit-up billboard everywhere she turned saying, "YOU ARE BROKEN."

In fact, she was far from broken. She, like you and me, had been guided away from everything true inside of her.

In her state of depression, which led to low energy levels, it was so easy for her to fall back into thought patterns that only made her feel worse. Further, it lead her to a lack of emotional fitness, which gives us the resourcefulness to pull ourselves out of bad states of mind and being.

She was caught in a pattern of judgment, lack, sadness, anger, and anxiety, and she couldn't get out.

This was all it was, a pattern—a pattern of thought, a pattern of focus that led to disempowering meaning being given to everything that had happened. She was living this story that was going to lead to a tragic ending.

I explained how, if she could just rewrite the story she was living, she could then change direction and have everything she wanted in life. For her, this was inner peace, self-love, passion for life, and freedom from those horrible beliefs that were slowly killing her.

I began working with this amazing athlete. I was so inspired by her determination to change her story, to change her life, and to do whatever was necessary to rewire her brain in a way that would see her celebrating how far she had come, rather than despairing over how far it seemed she had to go. She wanted to find deeper meaning and purpose. She wanted to find her true self and finally unchain from this version of herself that was built by the opinions, judgments, and beliefs of others.

Everything I have shared in this book, I started sharing with her. I took her through this entire process, step by step.

She went first in deciding she would NO LONGER live this story of being a woman afflicted with mental health issues whose life, relationships, and sense of self were falling apart.

She stopped saying "I am depressed," which had been her identity, and started saying, "I feel depressed," which was only temporary. This small shift enabled her to see that these feelings were just feelings. They were not who she was.

I had her write her new story, one that inspired her and empowered her.

She talked about living authentically and standing firm in the truth of who she was. She was an incredible human being who lived passionately, following her dreams and inspiring others to do the same. She was someone who was present in the beauty of this life and felt empowered knowing that her experience of life in every given moment was up to her. She cared deeply about animals and humans. She was going to make a difference in this world, and she was going to make THIS life everything she dreamed it to be.

She wrote her story and set up habits and rituals to condition this new story.

What would future her believe about what she was going through? What would future her do to feel better and to move beyond this rut she was in?

Future her would believe that this was a temporary state in which she had all the tools to get out of. Future her would believe that in overcoming this, she would become an even greater version of herself that could then take on any challenge and find a way through it, thriving on the other side. Future her would incorporate habits that would encourage this new way of thinking. She would discipline her focus so that it strengthened her, rather than weakened her. Future her would start to envision the future of what she wanted.

She would see herself grounded, centered, energized, living on purpose, and doing all the things that she dreamed of doing to the best of her ability. She would live from a place of flow, not force. She would celebrate her efforts, intentions, and commitments to living her best life in every moment.

She did all these things, every single day, catching herself when she inevitably would fall back into a painful, yet familiar pattern. She reminded herself that focusing on that negativity would not help her get to where she wanted to go. So, she would pivot, redirect her focus, and find a better way. The more she did this, it became habit, and it strengthened her. Each day, she built up her confidence and became the superhero of her own life in every moment.

She changed the channel from leading with love instead of fear. She lead with courage, presence, faith, intention, and authenticity.

Not only did she come out of this deep depression, but she also started training and racing again. I decided I would coach her as we had developed such an amazingly strong, trusting relationship. She is performing at higher levels than ever before. One of the most successful and dominant triathletes in the world.

I was more inspired to coach than ever before.

This time, though, it would be different. The mindset part would be the top priority and the swim, bike, and run secondary. We would be present for every step along this journey, as that was where the magic was.

The why would be to inspire others to believe in their own ability to overcome any challenge.

She would share her story to inspire others and help people who were floundering or struggling.

She would be the example of how to use your pain and struggles to touch other people's lives, as I have done through this book.

She became an agent of change, living proof, carrying all these principles I have shared with you and passing them on to others.

"With freedom comes responsibility."
— Eleanor Roosevelt

Pay it forward. Spread the word. Make this world a better place, one person at a time.

This is what it is all about.

I want you to share your story of how this book changed you, what it helped you overcome, and how different your life is now because of it.

You did the work. You took the leap and believed in me and most importantly, in YOU!

You now are an example and can share your story to help others FIND A WAY in their own lives.

My message for you when you are faced with hard times is to remind yourself and all those around you: DON'T POSTPONE JOY.

Find the joy and the magic moments amid the pain. If you look for it, you will find it.

In those moments where you are either trying to survive yourself or taking care of another person who needs you, DO NOT GIVE UP ON YOUR DREAMS.

If you give up on your dreams, you send out the energy that when things get hard, you jump ship, stay safe, withdraw, and sink.

Everything you do creates energy in the world.

What you do consistently becomes the pattern that touches every aspect of your life.

You are not a quitter. You are a warrior!

You don't give up. You lean in.

You don't live from fear. You live from love.

Which story do you choose to live?

This energy will touch every single challenge you face.

The above is my identity. I am someone that will ALWAYS FIND A WAY through any challenge. I am someone who will always find a way to achieve my dreams.

I am a WARRIOR.

I LEAN IN.

I live from a place of LOVE, not fear.

In the darkest moments of my illness, knowing who I am was what saved my life.

I knew that no matter how dark things got or how sick I was, I would find a way to triumph.

So will YOU!

You must EMBODY that belief, that attitude, that story.

You must KNOW this with all your being.

When you choose to be your highest, most beautifully powerful self, that energy fills those around you and they too learn to embody those characteristics.

Be the example of living authentically for your family and loved ones. Live in your truth, not your doubts. Live in your light, not your darkness. Live in your love, not your fear.

Shine your light brighter than ever before. It is when times are most dark that we must reach deeper within to find our own light so we can light the path for others.

Commit to this. Commit to you.

In taking care of yourself, you will discover how deeply this transforms the lives of all those around you.

It starts with you.

I believe in you.

I love you.

Siri

PART 3
Acknowledgments

To my wife, my superhero. This is for the countless hours, days, weeks, and months you fought hard to break through my stories and convince me that your love for me was real. There would be no change of heart. There would be no "other." You chose me. You fought for me. You showed me in every way, every day how much you love me. Thank you for bringing me strength and helping me see in myself what you see in me. Your love makes me feel like we can do anything we dream of. I know we will. You are my superwoman cape, and I love you with all my soul. You inspire me to be the very best me that I can be, every single day.

To my mom, forever my biggest cheerleader. Mom, you are the model for unconditional love. You pour your heart into everyone who has the gift of knowing you. I am always buoyed by your love and belief in me. I am inspired by the woman you are, chasing every dream you ever had and making it a reality. You overcome every great challenge with grace and fortitude. You treat your body like the temple it is, which sees you at eighty years old, climbing mountains, swimming across lakes, cycling for miles, and lifting the energy of any room you walk into.

You are my hero. Forever and always.

I will never forget a freezing cold day in Colorado. We were trying to muck the wet, muddy pasture behind the house. Every rake load was twenty pounds heavier due to the mud. Our hands were frozen, our feet were frozen, and we were exhausted, seemingly getting nowhere.

You turned to me and said, "At least there are no flies."

You were so right. In the summertime, we complained about the heat and the bucketloads of flies annoying the horses and biting welts into our legs. In those times, you say, "No frostbite."

Reframing is now one of my superpowers, and I know that came in large part from witnessing you do it all the time. Thank you. Thank you for being the most incredible mom any daughter could ask for. My rock. My best friend. I love you with all my soul.

Dad, I love watching you light up a room with your sense of humor, your easygoing nature, and your incredible storytelling.

What I have known for such a long time is that you love your own company. This has always been so inspiring to me. It gave me permission to love my own company.

You are the eternal optimist. You can find joy in the darkest of times and comfort in the worst situations. This is definitely a superpower. Thank you for coming back into my life and being the dad I always dreamed of. I am so sorry we missed out on so many years together. We won't focus on that, though; we will focus on the amazing memories we are creating now.

Thank you for being my biggest fan.

You have been the most incredible father to your sons, Kevin and Peter, my half-brothers.

One of the greatest blessings has been reconnecting with them with great hope in my heart that we will become closer and closer as the years go by.

In spending time with Kevin, it fills my heart to feel the similarities between us. Both of us have relished in your influence and are so grateful for it. What an extraordinary young man he is.

My sister, Lisa. I had a ton to live up to with you as my sister. You were absolutely brilliant, popular, adored, and the best athlete in high school. Being inspired by your greatness pushed me to do whatever I had to do to get good at the sports I loved. I wanted so much to be able to perform at the levels you did. This, I believe, was where my work ethic was born. I would study for hours and practice extra before and after team practices. I would rehearse things in my mind. I wanted to be as good as you. I wanted to make you proud of me. Thank you for pulling that out of me.

Your love is so pure. Your heart is so big. I am in awe of the love you bring out in others and how deeply they care after just moments in your presence. I am here for you, cheering you on as you face your toughest challenge yet.

You saved my life. The ultimate sacrifice and the most selfless gift.

Now it is time to save your own life.

We are here waiting with open arms and inspired hearts to welcome you home, healed and renewed. We are excited to share your second act, which will be full of love, joy, freedom, and fulfillment.

My Australian family. Second mum, Ruth, you have always been one of my biggest supporters. From the day I met you, I felt I had known you for a lifetime. Always so wise and so present, you are such a constant source of love and inspiration.

Simone, Bek's identical twin, what a gift it is to have you as a bonus sister, one who inspires me every single day. You are an incredible sister to Bek, and a fabulous mom to Charli and Milli. Thank you for letting me mistakenly squeeze your butt years ago and not shunning me for life. Instead, you laughed and made it a funny joke. I was so embarrassed.

Calvin, my angel forever. You came into my life at the perfect time. Sent from heaven, I am sure, you helped me find the strength to leave a situation that was slowly killing me. You then guided me down the path that would lead me to my mission and purpose. You were the most beautiful little man I have ever seen. I couldn't stop looking at you and into those soulful eyes that made me feel so safe, so seen, and so loved. I feel you with me always. The song of your soul plays on in my heart for eternity. You are my north star forevermore.

Savannah, my great teacher. My soulmate. My love. You challenge me every day to be the best version of myself. As I grow with you, I become more for others and for this world. Thank you for nourishing my soul and keeping me grounded in my truth always. I love you beyond words.

To all the animals that have blessed my life, every one of you left footprints in my heart and led me to who I am today. It is the ultimate gift to advocate for you. In advocating for you, we are advocating for the humans whose lives you have touched.

Gertie, Whoopi, Billy, Sophie, Athena, Buddha, Mabel, Millie, Lulu, Tulip, Zelda, Little Lady, Wonder, Grandpa, Grandma, Big Guy, Stormy, Heartsy, Duchess, Duke, Burt, Half-Pint, Eddie, Snickers, Moose, Posey, and the list goes on. You have touched me deeply, and I thank you for making the world a better place with your unconditional love and inspiration.

Tony Robbins, you are the most extraordinary man on this planet. I thank you for lighting the path for me over the last thirty years. Twenty years plus at Unleash the Power Within events, ten years plus at Date With Destiny events, and five years at Business Mastery events have given me the tools and strategies I needed to become the master of my emotions, mindset, and meaning. When you invited me to be a guest on your podcast, I thought you had made a mistake and were asking for one of my star athletes. But no, you wanted me. Who would have guessed that podcast, "How to Make the Decision to Do the Impossible," would end up being one of your most downloaded podcasts in history? It was the ultimate honor to be able to say thank you for having been such a huge influence on my life to that point. What happened next went beyond my wildest dreams. Thank you for asking me to share my story at these events that have shaped me and my entire life story. Thank you for choosing me to serve on this mission along with you. It is the most beautiful honor and privilege. In doing this work, I feel securely grounded in the knowledge that this is why I am here. Your belief in me gives me wings. Thank you. I love you so much.

Thank you, Sage Robbins and Mary Buckheit, for welcoming Bek and me into your extended family. For only having been in each other's lives for the last six years, I can't imagine a life without your beautiful family in it. Thank you for your love, friendship, guidance, and inspiration. You two remarkable women have changed my life in the most profound and glorious ways.

Melissa and Linda, our friendship is one of the most unexpected and incredible gifts. Thank you for going all in on this life together, bonded through love.

To Dr. Gutman, and Dr. Pollyea at UCHealth Anschutz, you are the most brilliant men I have ever met. Thank you for finding a way to not only save my life but to guide me to the other side stronger than ever before. I love you. Thank you.

Keri Anne, Taylor, Kate, Cynthia, and all the nurses and staff, thank you! You were my stars in the sky during my darkest nights. I couldn't have done this without you!

To all those who helped in my healing process: Sage, Mary, Dede, Jozee, Master Co, Brian, Scott, BioCharger, OsteoStrong, and of course, Tony.

To my umbilical cord donor, I hope to one day know who you are, so I can thank you personally. What a selfless and beautiful act of love to donate your umbilical cord to give life to another. I am forever grateful for this divine gift of life. Thank you so very much.

To all of you who prayed for me. To those who reached out on CaringBridge and GoFundMe, thank you. Love truly does heal.

To Mikey, Julia, and the entire UCHealth team filming my documentary, thank you for bringing this incredible story to life. I know it is going to help so many. I am so grateful for you.

To my entire family, thank you. Thank you, Auntie Karen, for being there for my mom, always. Thank you to my best friend, Loretta, always a pillar of strength for me. You are always an inspiration. I love you.

Thank you to all my friends, family, and clients who mean the world to me. You all hold a special place in my heart, and I am so deeply grateful for you. To my team at Keppler Speakers, Team Sirius Tri Club, 2Market Media, and Robbins Research International—thank you! To members of our Sirius Squad, Team Sirius Tri Club, Siriusly Authentic Squad, Etheridge Nation Warriors, and Go First to Success Squad, and all my current and former athletes, it is the ultimate privilege to guide you on this incredible journey to living your best lives.

To our Believe Ranch and Rescue and Horses in Our Hands family of supporters, thank you. We could not do the work we do without your support and love.

To Raoul, thank you for helping us keep our ranch thriving, magical, and safe. You are family to us, and we love you.

Katie, thank you for helping our gorgeous horses shine their lights by bringing out their magic through training.

Dr. Downey, thank you for always taking such beautiful care of our beloved horses.

Rachel, Jeanni, Mirinda, Ellie, Jen, Sean, Scott, Scarlett, Leah, Kaylin, Jill, and the amazing Becky Knott, I'm so grateful for you.

Thank you to my many teachers, mentors, and coaches. We are always learning; we are always growing. I am so deeply grateful to have learned, and continue to learn, from all of you. Coach Spellman, Tony, Sage, Mary, Carolyn, Wendy, Digit, Beth, Chris, Jackie, Lynn, Yoli, Jack, Jenny, Brett, Loretta, Sarah, Joseph, Scott, Diane, Lauren, Hank, Calvin, Savannah, Whoopi, Gertie, Mom, Dad, Ruth, and my amazing wife, Bek.

To Jan Miller, thank you for believing in me. I want so much to make you, Ali, Rebecca and Ivonne proud!

To Post Hill Press, thank you for being so incredible to work with. I feel so blessed to share this project with each and every one of you. Debra Englander my editor. Heather King and Caitlyn Limbaugh my managing editors. Alana Mills, production manager and Rachel Hoge, production editor. You are a world class team that I feel so proud to be a part of.

Thank you Gretchen. Thank you Beth. So grateful for you all.

Thank you to everyone who played a role in making this book happen. I am so deeply grateful you believed in me and in this book. It is my hope we will touch millions of lives with this creation.

To my friend Jeff Thrasher. I am so sad you didn't survive AML. You will be so missed. Everyday I commit to living life with all my heart and soul for you, and for all the other angels who found their wings.

To GOD. All glory be to you.

I am in awe of this miracle of life. I am forever grateful and committed to being all that you dream of me to be in this lifetime. Please, show me the way.

God, you are so good.

To my angels and my guides and this beautiful universe: Thank you.

Thank you.

Thank you.

To all of you:

Thank you for spending your precious time reading this book.

Thank you for believing in its ability to somehow move and inspire you.

I am grateful for you.

This book, my life's work, is for you.

May it be the gift and the blessing that I have intended.

To myself:

Siri, I love you.

I am so proud of you.

We did it!

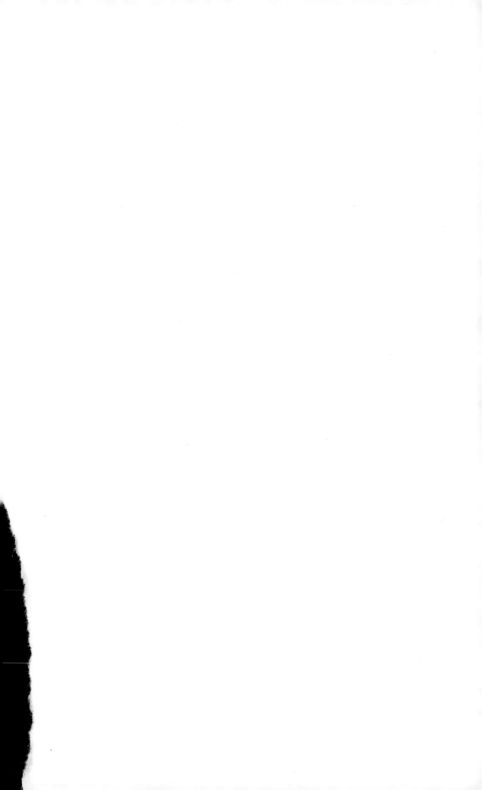

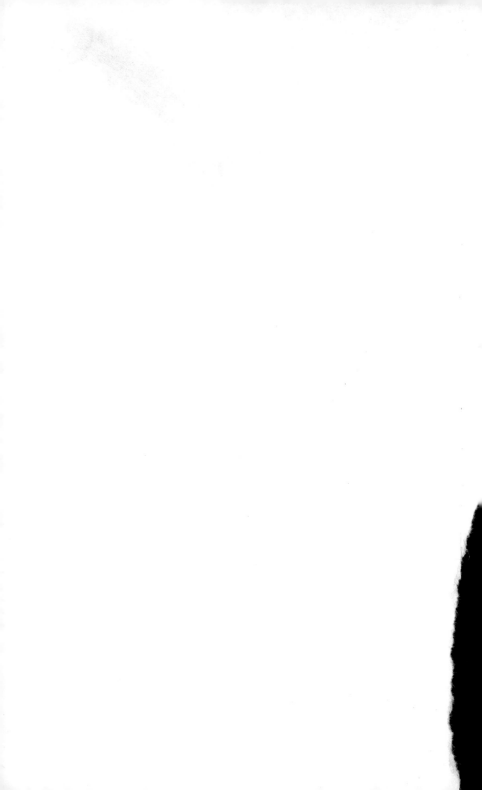